Principles of Science for Nurses

DATE DUE FOR RETURN

This book may be recalled before the above date.

PRINCIPLES OF SCIENCE FOR NURSES

Joyce James, Colin Baker & Helen Swain

Blackwell
Science

© 2002 by Blackwell Science Ltd
a Blackwell Publishing company

Editorial offices:
Blackwell Science Ltd, 9600 Garsington Road, Oxford
OX4 2DQ, UK
 Tel: +44 (0)1865 776868
Blackwell Publishing Inc., 350 Main Street,
Malden, MA 02148-5020, USA
 Tel: +1 781 388 8250
Blackwell Science Asia Pty, 550 Swanston Street,
Carlton, Victoria 3053, Australia
 Tel: +61 (0)3 8359 1011

First published 2002 by Blackwell Science Ltd.
Reprinted 2004

Library of Congress Cataloging-in-Publication Data
is available

ISBN 0-632-05769-6

A catalogue record for this title is available
from the British Library

Set in Souvenir
by SNP Best-set Typesetter Ltd., Hong Kong
Printed and bound in India using acid-free paper
by Replika Press Pvt. Ltd, Kundli 131028.

For further information on
Blackwell Publishing,visit our website:
www.blackwellpublishing.com

CONTENTS

PREFACE

The nursing profession has steadily developed from an untrained workforce to one that provides the highly skilled and educated nurses required in today's health service. Ever since Florence Nightingale started the first nursing school at St Thomas's Hospital the need for educated nurses has been recognised. The continued development of nursing education has seen nurses change from dependent to independent decision makers, a need which has become more important as specialist fields of expertise have evolved. A basic understanding of science and technology is vital to working effectively in this environment.

This book explains basic scientific concepts that are related to nursing practice. This will encourage and enable you to apply these concepts to your everyday working experience. Both the simplest and the most advanced practices and procedures have a fundamental underlying scientific principle. The ability to recognise this will provide a greater understanding of why things are done the way they are and should give you more confidence in contributing to the total care of your patients as well as enhancing your personal satisfaction and achievement.

A simple activity like giving a saline drip to restore fluid balance for example, could trigger a series of questions:

- Why does the fluid balance need restoring?
- Why is the bottle placed above the patient's head?
- What is normal saline?
- Why is it important to keep the lines sterile?

We hope to stimulate this spirit of enquiry in you.

There are a number of ways in which you may wish to use this book but as we recognise that you are not likely to study more than one chapter at a time, each chapter is designed to 'stand alone' as far as is possible. As you work through a chapter, activities and exercises are provided to encourage enquiry and test your understanding as you go. Simple and clear diagrams are provided where appropriate to support the explanations in the text. At the end of the chapter there are further questions to try, with answers provided.

There are several other important features. A glossary is provided which may be helpful for quick reference if there are terms in the text that you are uncertain about. At the start of this book important aspects of expressing measurements and the use of units have been summarised. These are essential for accurate reporting of the readings you have to record each day on the ward. Lastly, there are suggestions for further reading and some internet sites you can visit.

We wish you good luck with your studies!

Acknowledgements

Thank you to Lynn Jarvis for doing the graphics and to Deanne Cox our nurse advisor for all her help throughout the book.

INTRODUCTION

Homeostasis

Human beings are made up of millions of cells which are organised into tissues, organs and systems. The conditions inside the body are constantly changing as we break down food and synthesise molecules in response to particular situations. However, for each cell to function properly the fluid that surrounds the cell (extracellular fluid) and the fluid inside the cell (intracellular fluid) have to stay roughly the same. All the parts of the body work together to keep the extracellular and intracellular fluids as close as possible to the best or optimum conditions for the cell. The preservation of this internal environment of the body is called homeostasis.

There are only about 15 litres (L) of extracellular fluid (including blood) in the body, which has to cope with eliminating waste products and transporting nutrients to all of the cells within the body. Moreover, the concentrations of ions such as potassium and hydrogen within a cell have also to be maintained by transport into and out of the same fluids. An enormous task! It is easy to understand that the levels of all these factors will be constantly changing but must be quickly corrected to keep the extracellular fluid at an optimum for cell function. An uncorrected effect in an individual cell can quickly affect surrounding cells and ultimately loss of whole organ function and death.

Feedback mechanisms

Homeostasis can be thought of as a constantly self-adjusting or dynamic system which keeps the extracellular fluid within a fairly narrow range of parameters. This is made possible by a number of feedback mechanisms. Each feedback mechanism has three parts: a set point, a sensory receptor and an effector.

The set point is used as a reference to compare the fluid passing through it to the 'norm' for that fluid. Many set points are found in the hypothalamus which controls the release of hormones from the pituitary gland. The hypothalamus is connected to the pituitary gland and is located in the forebrain beneath the cerebral cortex. Sometimes the set point is referred to as an integrator because it receives information and selects different information, for the effectors, to bring about change (Fig. 0.1). One example is the control of body temperature; sensory receptors in the skin will respond to the environmental temperature and send a signal to the set point (integrator) in the brain The integrator responds by sending out signals to the muscles and glands which cause the correct response to maintain homeostasis.

This type of control is called negative feedback and is used by the body in hundreds of situations. Its effect is to cancel out the change (either less or more of a component) so that the levels are returned to the normal range.

The same kind of system is used to control the temperature of central heating, ovens and irons, when one part doesn't work the whole system is affected. Generally the speed at which homeostatic negative feedback occurs is not very fast, for example changes in blood glucose levels rely on the circulation of the blood to register that the glucose levels are not normal. They are also not corrected very accurately and overshooting the mark is common, which will have to be corrected again by the effectors. These reactions are automatic and self-adjusting: we cannot control them voluntarily.

Nurses need to realise that 'normal' levels will be within an acceptable range and should

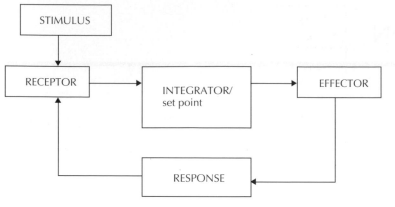

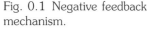

Fig. 0.1 Negative feedback mechanism.

be able to judge when changes occur. Taking the temperature of the patient is just one activity, which can indicate a homeostatic mechanism which is in or out of control.

Negative feedback control is used to control many different body functions which include respiration, breathing, and body temperature, but it is not the only type of control system, there are a few positive mechanisms as well.

Positive feedback increases an activity for a limited time to bring about a desired effect. A good example is the series of uterine contractions which expel the baby from the uterus in childbirth. This can be thought of as an unstable homeostatic state that lasts for a relatively short time. The fetus (stimulus) presses on the walls of the uterus and causes the pituitary gland to stimulate the production and secretion of oxytocin, which makes the muscles in the uterus wall contract, increasing the pressure on the fetus until it is expelled.

Many positive feedback mechanisms are harmful, e.g. cardiogenic shock (reduced blood flow to organs due to heart attack). During a heart attack less blood is circulated to the tissues, which become starved of oxygen. The tissues respond by changing their metabolism so that less oxygen is required. This leads to an increase in the volume of fluid bathing the cells (interstitial fluid) and a decrease in the volume of circulating blood. The positive feedback loop continues and makes the condition worse until

it becomes irreversible and death results (Fig. 0.2).

Unstable homeostatic states

When homeostatic mechanisms can no longer function, an unstable state or a stressed state predominates. Stress can be temporary (acute), e.g. injury or shock, or continual (chronic) as in long term disease. As we get older we become increasingly unable to respond to stress because our homeostatic mechanisms do not seem to function as well.

Many of the activities of a nurse are about restoring a homeostatic state to the patient who has become ill because they can no longer control their internal environment. Helping the patient to restore normal body temperature, fluid volume, chemical composition and electrolyte concentration, nutrients or the correct pH is a vital role for the nurse. Techniques and practices are constantly changing to accommodate new knowledge and better patient care but all have the same objective – to achieve the set point for the patient.

Measurement and units

Blood pressure, pulse, temperature, height and weight are a few of the measurements

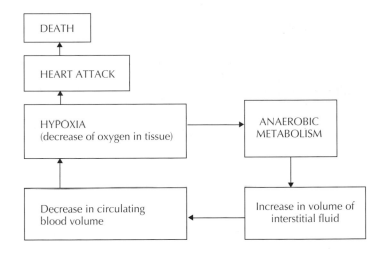

Fig. 0.2 Positive feedback – cardiogenic shock.

and recordings done by a nurse every day. There is always a need for accurate measurement and accurate recording. Records need to be interpreted by other staff so what is recorded must be clear and unambiguous. Continuous monitoring of a patient enables a good patient history to be built up and allows any changes in patient condition to be picked up early. It is equally important to understand measurements correctly in providing doses of medication.

Qualitative and quantitative measurement

There are three different types of measurement:

- **Qualitative** measurements are based on visual signs or the absence of signs but do not involve numbers. They rely on the observer's judgement so they are subjective.
- **Semi-qualitative** measurements record information on a relative scale. They are numerical estimates of an observation, for example a score of 5.3 in competitive ice-skating.
- **Quantitative** measurement – numbers are used to state the quantity which has been measured. This will normally require the use of an instrument to make the measurement. Examples are the measurement of height, weight, temperature and blood pressure. Most measurements of this type also require a unit to define the measurement. For example, it is not adequate to express body weight as 65 – do we mean pounds or kilograms? If it is kilograms then we must express the body weight as 65 kg to avoid any ambiguity! This type of measurement can be considered to be objective as it is based on a universally accepted scale.

An example of qualitative signs being converted to relative numerical values is the Apgar score used to indicate the condition of a new infant (Table 0.1).

A score is given for each of the five signs 1 and 5 minutes after the birth. A score of seven or above is considered satisfactory. Scores lower than seven indicate that some resuscitation may be required. In such cases, scores at subsequent 5-minute intervals would indicate the extent of recovery. In practice, the midwife will probably simply estimate the score without going through the whole process. Experience allows this to be done with accuracy.

Table 0.1 Apgar score

Sign	Score		
	0	1	2
Heart rate (beats min⁻¹)	Absent	Slow (below 100)	Over 100
Respiratory effort	Absent	Slow, irregular	Good, crying
Muscle tone	Flaccid	Some flexion of extremities	Active motion
Reflex irritability	No response	Grimace	Cough or sneeze
Colour	Blue, pale	Body pink, extremities blue	Completely pink

Recording numerical values

A few important points need to be borne in mind.

- When expressing values of less than one, the decimal point should always be preceded by a zero; hence 0.5 and not .5 should be written. This is simply a practical point to ensure clarity (in this case to avoid the number being read hurriedly as 5 which could be disastrous if it led to an error in drug dosage).
- You may be required to quote a value to 'so many' decimal places. This refers to the number of digits after the decimal place. So, 156.17 is quoted to two decimal places, 37.9 to one decimal place.
- The rule for rounding off to one less decimal place is that if the last number is 5 or more then add one to the previous decimal place, so 0.825 becomes 0.83 but 0.824 becomes 0.82.
- How the results of a measurement or calculation are expressed must reflect the accuracy of the least accurate individual measurement that has been taken. The concept of significant figures is used to indicate the numbers that are accurate. All non-zero numbers are significant but zeros at the end of a number are not unless they are followed by a decimal point. Look at the following simple calculations:

$200 \times 1.62 = 324$ but as the value 200 is only given to one significant figure, the answer should be given as 300!

$200.0 \times 1.62 = 324$ again and both 200.0 and 1.62 are given to three significant figures so this time the answer can be given as 324!

Units of measurement

As we saw above, when measuring (for example, mass, length or time) we need to indicate which system of units has been used for the measurement. The two common systems of units used in the United Kingdom are SI (Système International) and the more traditional imperial units. The simpler and more logical SI system is increasingly used in the hospital environment but there is a need to be aware of both types of units. For example, blood pressure is still quoted in mmHg. Conversion from one system to another can be achieved using conversion tables or simple conversion formulae. Some commonly used conversion factors are given in Table 0.2:

So for example to convert 1 pound (16 ounces) into grams you simply multiply 16 by the conversion factor (28.35) to give 453.6 g.

Table 0.2 Conversion to SI units

Non-SI unit	Equivalent SI unit	Conversion factor
pound (lb)	kilogram (kg);	0.454
yard	metre (m);	0.914
ounce (oz)	gram (g)	28.359
mm Hg (pressure)	pascal (Pa)	133.30
pounds per square inch (psi)	pascal (Pa)	6895.156
calorie	joule (J)	4.184

Table 0.3 Base units

Quantity	SI unit
length	metre (m)
mass	kilogram (kg)
time	second (s)
current	ampere (A)
temperature	kelvin (K)
amount of substance	mole (mol)

Table 0.4 Common derived units

Physical Quantity	SI unit
force	newton (N)
energy	joule (J)
pressure	pascal (Pa)
potential difference	volt (V)
frequency	hertz (Hz)
volume	cubic metres (m^3)

Exercise 0.1

Convert:
a)   75 pounds to kilograms
b)   110 yards to metres
c)   1500 calories to joules
Express each answer to two significant figures.

A distinction is sometimes made between base (fundamental) and derived units, the latter are units of quantity that require the measurement of more than one of the base units. Examples are given in Tables 0.3 and 0.4.

Expressing derived units

There are a number of different ways we can write some derived units. You should be aware of their equivalence. For example, speed (calculated as distance divided by time) can be written in each of the following ways: metres per second, m/s or ms^{-1}. The reciprocal index ($^{-1}$) is used to indicate that time (s) is the divisor. Similarly, pressure can be expressed as newtons per square metre or N/m^2 or Nm^{-2}.

Dealing with large and small numbers

In science we often have to deal with very large or very small numbers. For example the number of particles in a mole is approximately 600 000 000 000 000 000 000 000, X-rays have a wavelength of about 0.000 000 000 01 metres! These are very cumbersome numbers to write down and it would be difficult to ensure you wrote down exactly the right number of noughts.

Expressing these sorts of numbers is far easier in the standard form based on the use of indices. Consider multiples of 10:

$$100 \quad = 10 \times 10$$
$$= 10^2$$
$$1000 \quad = 10 \times 10 \times 10$$
$$= 10^3$$
$$10\,000 \quad = 10 \times 10 \times 10 \times 10$$
$$= 10^4$$
$$100\,000 \quad = 10 \times 10 \times 10 \times 10 \times 10$$
$$= 10^5$$
$$1\,000\,000 = 10 \times 10 \times 10 \times 10 \times 10 \times 10$$
$$= 10^6$$

and so on. Note that the figure above the ten ('ten to the power of' or the index) is equal to the number of zeros in the number written out longhand and the number of times 10 is multiplied by itself. Hence:

$$2500 \quad = 2.5 \times 1000 \quad = 2.5 \times 10^3$$
$$697\,000 = 6.97 \times 100\,000 = 6.97 \times 10^5$$

and we have a convenient and compact way of dealing with these types of figures.

Small numbers (less than 1)

Numbers with a value of less than one can be expressed as follows, using the reciprocal index:

$$0.1 \qquad 1/10 \qquad = 1.0 \times 10^{-1}$$
$$0.01 \qquad 1/100 \qquad = 1.0 \times 10^{-2}$$
$$0.001 \qquad 1/1000 \qquad = 1.0 \times 10^{-3}$$
$$0.0037 \qquad 37/1000 \qquad = 3.7 \times 10^{-3}$$
$$0.000\,007\,3 \quad 73/1\,000\,000 = 7.3 \times 10^{-6}$$

The negative sign in front of the index value indicates that the power of ten is dividing and not multiplying the given digit. As a rule of thumb, the index value indicates the number of places the decimal place has been moved to the left.

Exercise 0.2

Numbers written in the form 1.7×10^3 and 9.26×10^{-5} are said to be written in the standard form. Express the following numbers in the standard form:
a) 0.000 000 000 5
b) 301 000 000
c) 78 100 000
d) 128 400

Prefixes for SI units

When dealing with multiples and submultiples of the basic SI units, the prefixes in Table 0.5 are used. Since a lot of measurements associated with the body and medication are very small, a correct understanding and use of these prefixes is very important.

Simple conversions in SI units only require the use of the prefixes for multiples and submultiples.

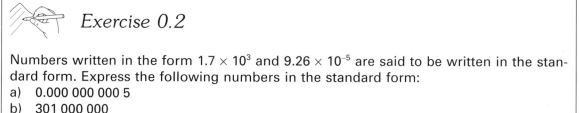

kilogram — Multiply by 1000 (10^3) → gram — Multiply by 1000 (10^3) → milligram
kilogram ← Divide by 1000 (10^3) — gram ← Divide by 1000 (10^3) — milligram

Table 0.5 Prefixes for SI units

Prefix	Symbol	Multiple	Standard notation
mega	M	one million	10^6
kilo	k	one thousand	10^3
deci	d	one tenth	10^{-1}
centl	c	one hundredth	10^{-2}
milli	m	one thousandth	10^{-3}
micro	mc	one millionth	10^{-6}
nano	n	one thousand millionth	10^{-9}

So, 1 **kilo**gram = 1000 grams
  1 **milli**gram = 10^{-3} gram (0.001 gram)

To convert from milligrams to micrograms, the table above indicates that there are 10^3 micrograms in 1 milligram (why?), so 1000 or 10^3 is the factor for this conversion. One point to note is that in scientific notation a microgram is abbreviated to µg. However for greater clarity in nursing work the abbreviation mcg or the full name should be used.

Measuring volumes

Although the cubic metre is the correct SI unit of volume the most commonly used metric measurement of volume is the litre (L) or millilitre (mL). One litre is equal to $1000\,cm^3$ so you can see that $1\,cm^3$ is also equivalent to $1\,mL$. It may also be useful to know that a litre is approximately equal to 0.11 gallons and 2.2 pints.

Exercise 0.3

Express:
a) 1×10^{-6} g in micrograms (mcg)
b)   474 joules as kilojoules (kJ)
c)   700 millilitres (mL) as litres (L)

Percentages, fractions and ratios

These can be used to express the same information in a variety of forms. The term 'per cent' means 'in each hundred' so a percentage value expresses the number of parts in a hundred parts of whatever is being measured. Hence if we state that 4% of the population have the AB blood group we are saying that four in every hundred people have that type of blood. The same statistic can be expressed as a fraction – 4/100 that we can simplify to 1/25 by dividing both numbers in the fraction by four. This fraction can be converted back to a percentage by multiplying the fraction by 100. The general equation for calculating a percentage is:

Percentage value
$$= \frac{\text{value of item being measured}}{\text{total number of items in system}} \times 100$$

Ratios can be also used to express quantities in a similar way: 4% can also be expressed as the ratio $4:96$. In this case we are saying that there are 4 people with the AB blood group to every 96 people with other blood groups in a population of 100. Ratios can be simplified in the same way as fractions by dividing each value by the same factor. So, $1:25$ states the same ratio as $4:96$ or 4%.

Percentages and ratios are often used in describing the concentration of solutions. Hence a 1% solution of sodium citrate contains one part of sodium citrate (the solute) in a hundred parts of solution. The value is independent of the units of measurement. So, 5 g citric acid in 250 g of solution would be described by the following percentage:

$$\frac{5}{250} \times 100 = 2\%$$

2 kg (2000 g) of this 2% solution would contain $2000 \times 2/100 = 40$ g sodium citrate.

You may also find very low concentrations described in parts per million (ppm). A 1 ppm solution contains one part of solute dissolved in one million parts of solution.

Exercise 0.4

a) Change these fractions to percentages: 3/5, 17/20, 9/25
b) Change these ratios to the form 1 in 'x' and then write as percentages: $1:24$, $1:9$, $1:40$

Many simple drug calculations can be worked out by using the formula below which uses the fraction of the dose required provided by each measure (pill, spoonful or solution of known concentration) to identify the number of measures to be given.

Number of measures to be given

$$= \frac{\text{dose prescribed}}{\text{dose per measure}}$$

For example, a patient is ordered 0.25 mg of digioxin, orally. The digioxin available is in tablets containing 125 micrograms (mcg). First we have to recognise that we *must* be consistent with our units – the 0.25 mg dose prescribed is equivalent to 250 mcg. Then, substituting the values in the formula:

Number of measures to be given

$$= \frac{\text{dose prescribed}}{\text{dose per measure}} = \frac{250}{125} = 2 \text{ tablets}$$

Exercise 0.5

An injection of morphine 8 mg is required. Ampoules available contain 10 mg in 2 ml. What volume is drawn up for injection? Hint: use the formula above, the fraction produced will be the fraction of the ampoule required.

Averages

Averages allow you to express a series of values or readings as a single, meaningful value. The most common type of average value is the mean. It is worked out as follows:

$$\text{Mean} = \frac{\text{sum of all the readings}}{\text{number of readings taken}}$$

For example, the seven nurses on a ward have ages of 22, 26, 30, 32, 33, 39 and 51 respectively. The average (mean) age is:

$$\frac{22 + 26 + 30 + 32 + 33 + 39 + 51}{7} = 33$$

We might also quote the median, the middle value in the range of figures. This is 32 in this case, not necessarily the same as the mean value.

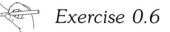

Exercise 0.6

Calculate the average weekly temperature (°C) of a patient from the following data. To how many decimal places should you express your answer?

Mon	Tues	Wed	Thurs	Fri	Sat	Sun
36.4	36.8	37.0	37.1	37.5	37.9	36.9

Graphs and conversion charts

Numerical information is often conveniently presented in graphs or conversion charts. In Fig. 0.3 the data from the exercise above have been plotted graphically; time (days of the week) on the x-axis and temperature on the y-axis. This type of presentation of data enables us to see trends at a glance as well as take readings directly from the graph. For example, the value plotted for Wednesday's temperature is simply read off on the y-axis as 37.0°C. It can immediately be seen that the patient's temperature rose steadily until Saturday and then dropped back down again.

Summary

- Quantitative measurements are based on numerical figures, qualitative measurement on other visual signs

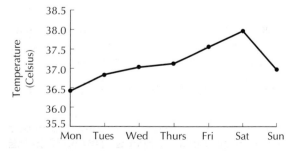

Fig. 0.3 Temperature plotted against time.

- The SI system of units has now largely replaced the 'older' imperial measures. If required, interconversion between these units can be achieved using simple conversion factors
- The 'standard form' is important in expressing large and small quantities in a convenient way. The use of prefixes to SI units can be used to achieve the same aim
- Percentages, fractions and ratios can be readily and simply interconverted
- Averages can provide a single meaningful figure to represent a series of measurements
- The graphical representation of data is a useful and convenient way of presenting information.

Review questions

1. Steve Jones cycles to work every morning. His resting pulse rate is $72\,min^{-1}$ but when he arrives at work this has increased to $81\,min^{-1}$. What is the percentage increase in his pulse rate?

2. Blood makes up 7% of the body weight. If each of the following people donated one pint of blood, what percentage of their blood has each person given:
    (a) Polly   50 kg
    (b) Joyce   10 stone
    1 pint of blood weighs 600 g; 1 stone = 6.35 kg

3.   A patient requires 1.250 g of an antibiotic that is supplied in tablet form, each containing 250 mg of the antibiotic. How many tablets are needed for the correct dose?

4.   Fig. 0.4 illustrates the effect of drinking 1 L of water on the rate of urine production. From the graph, state the time in minutes that the maximum amount of urine is produced. After 120 min, what is the volume of urine being produced?

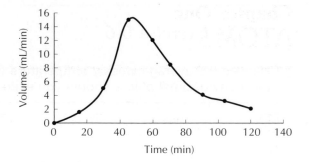

Fig. 0.4 Urine production plotted against time.

Chapter One
ATOMS

Learning objectives

By the end of the chapter the reader will be able to:
- Identify the states of matter
- Describe the structure of the atom in terms of electrons, protons and neutrons
- Define the terms element, molecule, ion, radical, compound, atomic number, mass number and isotope
- List the main elements contained in the body
- Explain how ionic and covalent bonds are formed
- Distinguish between polar and non-polar molecules
- Explain the concept of the mole.

Introduction

Atoms, the compounds they form and the chemical reactions which they undergo form the basis of life. All living creatures (and that includes you!) are essentially a collection of atoms – a very complex and organised collection of atoms, but still atoms. Any understanding of human physiology must therefore go hand in hand with an understanding of the amazing atom.

Matter

Everything in the universe is made up of matter. Matter is anything that occupies space and has mass. All matter is made up of particles. There are three states of matter: solid, liquid and gas (Fig. 1.1).

Changes of state

When a solid is heated it changes state and forms a liquid. If you continue to heat the liquid, then it will change state again, to form a gas. Some substances can go from the solid state to the gaseous state directly, for example iodine, this is known as sublimation.

All particles possess kinetic energy (energy of movement). Solid particles have a small amount of kinetic energy, liquid particles more and gas particles the most. Changes of state always involve the addition or removal of energy, normally in the form of heat (Figs 1.2 & 1.3).

The core body temperature, in humans, is 37°C. Body temperature is altered by illness, exercise or climatic changes. One of the mechanisms for maintaining body temperature is sweating. Up to 12 L of water a day can be lost through sweating. Sweat evaporates from the surface of the skin cooling the body. Heat is removed from the body by changing the state of sweat from a liquid to a gas.

State	Arrangement of Particles	
SOLID	Solids have a definite shape and volume. Very strong forces of attraction between particles. Particles only vibrate about a point. Solids are rigid.	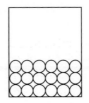
LIQUID	Liquids flow. They have a definite volume, but their shape depends on the container. Weak forces of attraction between the particles. Particles move and slide over each other.	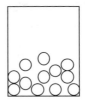
GAS	Gases flow. Gases have no definite volume or shape and they fill all the space available. Almost no forces of attraction between particles. Particles move in a random manner colliding with other particles and the walls of the container.	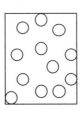

Fig. 1.1 States of matter.

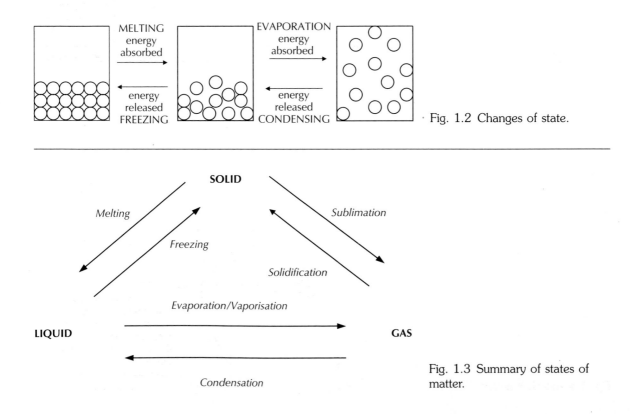

Fig. 1.2 Changes of state.

Fig. 1.3 Summary of states of matter.

Atoms

About 2500 years ago a Greek philosopher called Democritus suggested that all matter in the universe is made up of tiny, indivisible particles. In 1807 John Dalton called these tiny particles 'atoms', from the Greek word *atomos* meaning indivisible. We now know that atoms are not indivisible, the nuclear or atomic bomb being the result of splitting the atom. However the atom still remains the smallest particle that can exist independently and the smallest unit that can enter a chemical reaction.

Atoms are approximately $1/100\,000\,000$ of a centimetre across; 100 million atoms side by side would therefore measure 1 cm (Fig. 1.4).

Atomic structure

Atoms are made up of protons, neutrons and electrons – these are called sub-atomic particles (Fig. 1.5).

The central nucleus contains protons and neutrons. The mass of the atom is concentrated in the central nucleus and is very small. Moving around the nucleus are electrons. The electrons are arranged in orbitals or shells or energy levels at different distances from the nucleus. The mass of the electron is so small it can be ignored when working out the mass

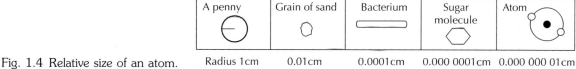

A penny	Grain of sand	Bacterium	Sugar molecule	Atom
Radius 1cm	0.01cm	0.0001cm	0.000 0001cm	0.000 000 01cm

Fig. 1.4 Relative size of an atom.

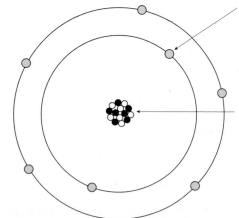

ELECTRONS
- Move around the nucleus, in shells
- Are negatively charged
- Are very small
- Have virtually no mass

NUCLEUS
- Is in the centre of the atom
- Contains protons and neutrons
- Protons are positively charged, neutrons have no charge
- The nucleus has a positive overall charge
- The mass of the atom is within the nucleus

Fig. 1.5 Atomic structure.

of the atom. Chemical reactions involve only electrons (Table 1.1).

▪ ▪ Elements

An element is a substance in which all the atoms have the same chemical properties. Over 100 elements exist. A Russian scientist called Dmitri Mendeléev conveniently arranged these into a table called the periodic table (Fig. 1.6 & p. 227). He arranged the elements in horizontal rows – periods and vertical columns – groups. It is called the periodic table since the structure and chemical reactivity of the elements arranged in the rows, or periods, show repeating or periodic characteristics.

Each element in the periodic table is represented by a symbol. Most elements have two letters in their symbol; the first letter is a capital, and the second letter is *always* small. If there is only one letter this is always a capital. These symbols come from either the English name (C for carbon) or the Latin (Na for natrium, English sodium; K for kalium, English potassium). Medical terminology often uses Latin terms so hypernatraemia and hyperkalaemia are used to indicate high levels of sodium and potassium in the body.

Table 1.1 Sub-atomic particles

Particle	Position	Mass (relative to that of a proton)	Charge (relative to that on a proton)
Proton	Nucleus	1	+1
Neutron	Nucleus	1	0
Electron	Shells	$\frac{1}{1840}$	−1

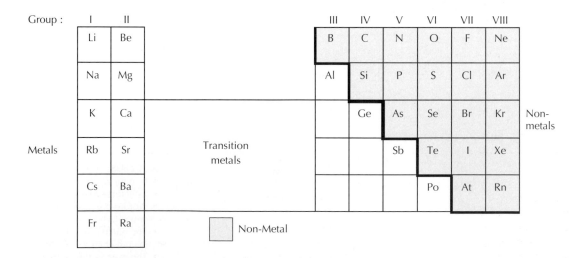

Fig. 1.6 Abridged periodic table, showing groups, metals and non-metals.

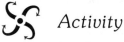 *Activity*

Using the periodic table provided on p. 227 find the symbols that represent the following elements:

Element	Symbol
Mercury	
Iron	
Gold	
Lead	

Classification of the elements

Elements can be conveniently divided into two broad categories; metals and non-metals. This can be done on the basis of their properties (Table 1.2).

Metals are found on the left-hand side of the periodic table, e.g. sodium and calcium and non-metals are found on the right-hand side, e.g. oxygen and chlorine.

Elements in the body

The number of elements found in the body is small. In fact 95% of a living organism is made up of only four elements – carbon, oxygen, hydrogen and nitrogen (Fig. 1.7).

Trace elements for example, iron (Fe), iodine (I), copper (Cu), chromium (Cr) and zinc (Zn) are

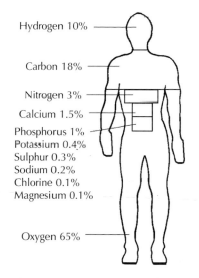

Hydrogen 10%
Carbon 18%
Nitrogen 3%
Calcium 1.5%
Phosphorus 1%
Potassium 0.4%
Sulphur 0.3%
Sodium 0.2%
Chlorine 0.1%
Magnesium 0.1%
Oxygen 65%

Fig. 1.7 Elements in the body.

Table 1.2 Classification of the elements

Property	Metals	Non-metals
physical state	solid (except mercury)	solid, liquid or gas
lustre	shiny	dull
boiling point/melting point	high	low
conductors of heat/electricity	good	poor, good insulators
affinity for electrons	donates electrons	accepts electrons

needed in very small quantities by the body. Many are found as parts of enzymes or are needed for enzyme activity. In excess they can be toxic.

Toxic elements e.g. mercury (Hg), lead (Pb), arsenic (As) and thallium (Tl) can all cause death, their toxic effect is cumulative.

Activity

Mercury is a toxic element and can lead to death. In hospitals it is commonly used in thermometers and sphygmomanometers. Look up the symptoms of mercury poisoning and the type of treatment given to such a patient.

Atomic number and mass number

The atomic number is the number of protons that the atom contains (Fig. 1.8). In a neutral atom, this is also the same as the number of electrons. The elements are arranged in order of their increasing atomic number in the periodic table.

The mass number is the number of protons, plus the number of neutrons (Fig. 1.8). The mass number is always larger, roughly twice the size of the atomic number.

Isotopes

Isotopes are atoms of the same element that have the same atomic number but different mass numbers. Isotopes have a different

numbers of neutrons in their nucleus. For example iodine:

	$^{123}_{54}I$	$^{125}_{54}I$	$^{127}_{54}I$	$^{131}_{54}I$
protons	54	54	54	54
electrons	54	54	54	54
neutrons	69	71	73	77

Isotopes which are radioactive are called radioisotopes. These are covered in more detail in Chapter 11. Isotopes can be written as either ^{131}I or iodine-131.

Isotopes have the same chemical properties, since this is dependent on the number of electrons in an atom, but they will have different physical properties (e.g. boiling and melting points) as their masses are different.

The element iodine is essential for the production of the hormone thyroxine by the thyroid gland. Radioactive iodine-131 is used as a diagnostic test for hyperthyroidism (overactive thyroid), e.g. Graves disease, or hypothyroidism (myxoedema – underactive thyroid) and thyroid cancer. The patient is given a solution of sodium iodide containing a small amount (trace) of iodine-131. The quantity of iodine-131 absorbed by the thyroid gland or excreted in the urine is measured using a gamma detector.

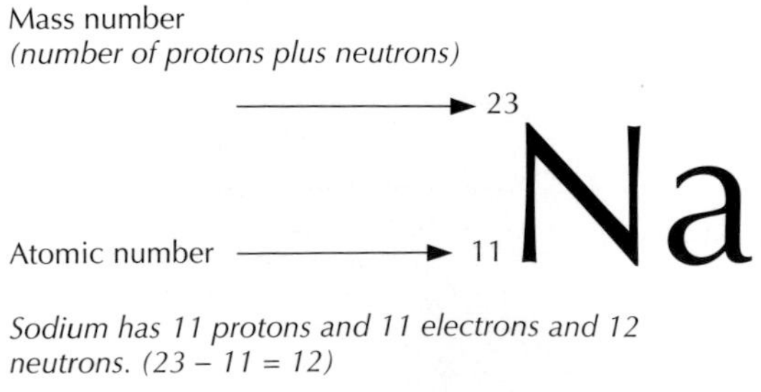

Relative atomic mass

An atom of the carbon-12 isotope was given a relative atomic mass of 12.0000 u (u = atomic

Mass number
(number of protons plus neutrons)

$$^{23}_{11}Na$$

Atomic number

Sodium has 11 protons and 11 electrons and 12 neutrons. (23 − 11 = 12)

Fig. 1.8 Atomic and mass numbers.

mass unit). The relative masses of all other atoms were then obtained by comparison to this standard atom. The relative atomic mass is also called 'atomic mass', 'average atomic mass' and in the past 'atomic weight'.

Most elements contain a mixture of isotopes. The relative atomic mass of an element is the average mass of one atom, taking account of all its isotopes and their relative proportions compared with an atom of carbon-12.

For example chlorine consists of two isotopes with mass numbers of 35 and 37. These isotopes are written as chlorine-35 and chlorine-37 respectively. Naturally occurring chlorine contains 75% of chlorine-35 and 25% of chlorine-37. The relative atomic mass of chlorine is:

$$\frac{(75 \times 35) + (25 \times 37)}{100} = 35.5 \text{ u}$$

Most relative atomic masses are not whole numbers because most elements have many isotopes (Table 1.3).

Electron arrangement

Electrons are arranged in shells around the nucleus. The number of electrons in a neutral atom is given by the atomic number. The rules for filling the shells are:

Table 1.3 The relative atomic masses of some elements

Element	Symbol	Relative atomic mass
Carbon	C	12.011
Hydrogen	H	1.008
Magnesium	Mg	24.312
Sodium	Na	22.989
Sulphur	S	32.064

1. The shell nearest the nucleus fills first
2. Only a given number of electrons are allowed in each shell

Examples

1st shell 2 2nd shell 8 3rd shell 18

The diagrams like those in Figs 1.9 and 1.10 are quite cumbersome to draw each time, so a shorthand form is often used to show how electrons are arranged – this is called the electronic configuration.

- The electronic configuration for carbon is written as   C 2, 4
- The electronic configuration for sodium is written as   Na 2, 8, 1

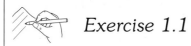 *Exercise 1.1*

The atomic number of lithium is 3. Draw a diagram to show the electronic arrangement and write the electronic configuration for this atom.

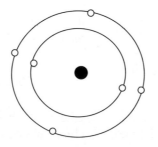

CARBON – atomic number 6
It has 6 electrons,
2 occupy the first shell (making it full),
leaving 4 in the second shell.

Fig. 1.9 Electronic arrangement of carbon.

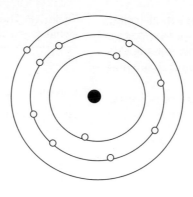

SODIUM – atomic number 11
It has 11 electrons,
2 occupy the first shell (making it full),
8 occupy the second shell (making it full),
leaving 1 in the third shell.

Fig. 1.10 Electronic arrangement of sodium.

Compounds

Jilly was a chemist, but Jilly is no more,
For, what she thought was H_2O, was H_2SO_4.

A compound is a substance that contains two or more elements joined together by a chemical bond (Table 1.4). The property of the compound will usually be very different from those of the individual elements in it,

e.g.   sodium   +   chlorine   →   sodium
       reacts   *corrosive*   chloride
       violently   *gas*   (table salt)
       with water   *nice with*
                                chips,
                                yummy!

Table 1.4 Simple compounds

Name of compound	Elements found and their symbols	How the atoms join up (structural formula)	Formula of compound
Water	Hydrogen (H) and oxygen (O)	H–O–H	H_2O
Carbon monoxide	Carbon (C) and oxygen (O)	C≡O	CO
Ethanol (alcohol)	Carbon (C) and oxygen (O) and hydrogen (H)	$H-CH_2-CH_2-OH$	C_2H_5OH
Ammonia	Nitrogen (N) and hydrogen (H)	H–N–H ⎪H	NH_3

Compounds are generally named after the elements that reacted to form them. A shorthand way of describing a compound is by writing its name as a chemical formula. The formula of a compound indicates the number and type of each atom present, e.g. carbon dioxide contains one carbon atom and two oxygen atoms (indicated by the prefix 'di') and its formula is CO_2 (note the number 2 is written as a subscript).

Chemical equations

Chemical equations are a way of representing chemical changes which occur when elements or compounds react together. They tell us what substances are reacting together – (reactants) and what new substances are formed – (products). Equations can be in the form of words or symbols.

There are three stages in writing an equation:

- Write a word equation for the reaction

  hydrogen + oxygen $\rightarrow$ water

- Write the formulae for the reactants and products. The symbol (s) after the formula indicates solid; (l) is used for liquid; (g) for gas and (aq) for an aqueous solution (i.e. a substance dissolved in water).

  $H_{2(g)} + O_{2(g)} \rightarrow H_2O_{(l)}$

- Balance the equation by making the number of atoms of each element the same on both sides as you cannot create or destroy matter.

  $2H_{2(g)} + O_{2(g)} \rightarrow 2H_2O_{(l)}$

The large 2 in front of the hydrogen and the water means that you must multiply all the atoms in the formula by 2, i.e. 2 (H_2) = 4 hydrogen atoms; 2 (H_2O) = 4 hydrogen atoms and 2 oxygen atoms. The numbers in front of the formulae indicate the ratio in which they react or are formed.

A single headed arrow $\rightarrow$ indicates that all or nearly all the reactants will become products. The arrow indicates the direction of the reaction, this reaction has gone from left to right (forward reaction). Just as when you bake a cake once you have mixed the ingredients and baked them in the oven you cannot get back your starting ingredients – the reaction is irreversible.

Double arrows $\rightleftarrows$ indicate a reversible reaction. In a reversible reaction the reaction can go in both directions, that is the reactants go to products and the products go back to reactants. For example ice turns to water on heating but on cooling it becomes ice again:

$H_2O_{(ICE)} \rightleftarrows H_2O_{(WATER)}$

An example of a reversible reaction in the body is the reaction between haemoglobin and oxygen:

Hb + O_2 $\rightleftarrows$ HbO_2
haemoglobin oxygen oxyhaemoglobin

In a reversible reaction when the rate of the forward reaction (left to right) equals the rate of the backward reaction (right to left), a balance between products and reactants exists. This is known as an equilibrium reaction. Two half arrows $\rightleftarrows$ indicate an equilibrium reaction. It is a dynamic situation since reactants are continually changing to products and products back to reactants. However the concentration or amount of reactants and products always remains the same at equilibrium at a given set of conditions. In the human body the conditions at equilibrium are 37 °C and atmospheric pressure.

So if ice and water are kept at 0 °C, neither the ice nor the water seems to change since the two substances are in equilibrium and we can write:

$H_2O_{(ICE)} \rightleftarrows H_2O_{(WATER)}$

Similarly with haemoglobin an equilibrium reaction exists in the body;

Hb + O_2 $\rightleftarrows$ HbO_2
haemoglobin oxygen oxyhaemoglobin

Equilibrium reactions are very important in maintaining homeostatic conditions in the body. When a person is ill, conditions in the body change and this can alter the position of the equilibrium. The most important change in physiological systems is change in concentration of reactants and products. The effects of changing conditions on an equilibrium can be predicted using Le Chatelier's principle. It states that if an equilibrium is disturbed by changing conditions, the reaction moves to counteract the change.

If we look at the haemoglobin system again:

$\Leftarrow$ low levels of oxygen in tissue, equilibrium moves to the left, to increase the oxygen concentration.

$$Hb + O_2 \rightleftharpoons HbO_2$$

$\Rightarrow$ high levels of oxygen in tissue, equilibrium moves to the right, to decrease the oxygen concentration.

When the concentration of oxygen in the body is decreased, as for example in the tissues, the equilibrium will change to compensate for this. The equilibrium will move to the left, so the concentration of oxyhaemoglobin in the equilibrium will decrease but the concentration of oxygen will increase.

If the concentration of oxygen is increased as for example in the lungs then the equilibrium will move to the right, so the concentration of oxyhaemoglobin increases and the concentration of oxygen will decrease.

This type of balancing act ensures that oxyhaemoglobin releases oxygen to tissues when needed and also that haemoglobin picks up oxygen when there is a plentiful supply of oxygen.

Chemical bonding

Compounds are substances that consist of atoms joined together by chemical bonds. Chemical reactions involve changes in the number of electrons atoms have.

The Noble or inert gases are found in Group 8 of the periodic table. They are different from other elements because they do not usually form compounds. Their atoms are unreactive or stable. They are stable because their outer electron shells contain 2 or 8 electrons, hence the Noble gases exist as atoms, whilst all other gases are molecules (Fig. 1.11).

All other atoms have partially filled outer shells – this is why they react. Atoms react with each other to obtain a full outer shell so they can become stable.

Ionic bonds – losing or gaining electrons to obtain a full outer shell

Ionic bonds are formed between metal atoms and non-metal atoms. Ions are formed. Ions are charged particles and are formed when an atom loses or gains an electron.

Losing electrons

Metals obtain their full outer shell by losing their outermost electrons to a non-metal atom. The result of losing an electron is the formation of

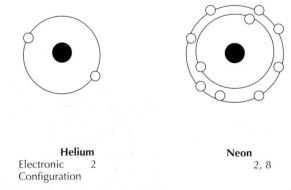
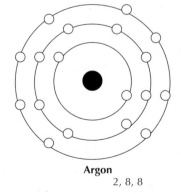

| | Helium | Neon | Argon |
| Electronic Configuration | 2 | 2, 8 | 2, 8, 8 |

Fig. 1.11 Electronic structure of noble gases.

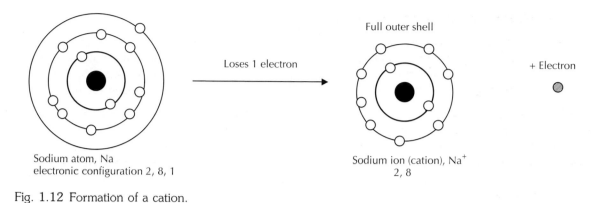

Sodium atom, Na
electronic configuration 2, 8, 1

Sodium ion (cation), Na⁺
2, 8

Full outer shell

Loses 1 electron

+ Electron

Fig. 1.12 Formation of a cation.

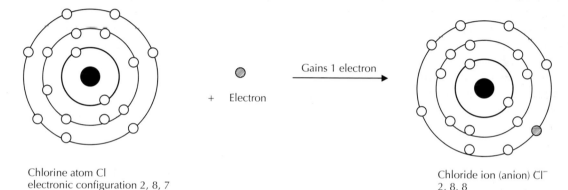

Chlorine atom Cl
electronic configuration 2, 8, 7

+   Electron

Gains 1 electron

Chloride ion (anion) Cl⁻
2, 8, 8

Fig. 1.13 Formation of an anion.

a positively charged ion called a cation. For example sodium has one electron in its outer shell, it obtains its full outer shell by losing this electron forming a cation (Fig. 1.12).

A sodium atom has 11 electrons and 11 protons. The sodium ion has 11 protons and 10 electrons, so it has a single positive charge since it has 'lost' an electron.

Gaining an electron

Non-metals obtain their full outer shell by accepting electrons. A negatively charged ion called an anion is formed. For example, chlorine has seven electrons in its outside shell, it obtains a full shell by accepting an electron and forming an anion (Fig. 1.13).

A chloride atom has 17 electrons and 17 protons. The chloride ion has 17 protons and 18 electrons, so it has a single negative charge since it has 'gained' an electron.

The reaction between sodium and chlorine

When sodium, a metal, reacts with chlorine, a non-metal, the sodium atom loses its electron to the chlorine atom. For clarity in Fig. 1.14 the electrons are represented by ◉ and ○ but all the electrons are exactly the same.

Therefore in an ionic bond two ions are formed, a positive cation and a negative anion. Opposites charges attract and it is the

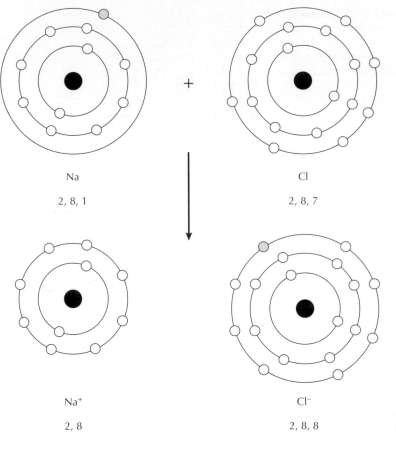

Na

2, 8, 1

Cl

2, 8, 7

Na$^+$

2, 8

Cl$^-$

2, 8, 8

Fig. 1.14 The formation of sodium chloride.

force of attraction between the cation and the anion that forms the ionic bond or electrovalent bond.

The number of electrons lost by the metal atom is its valency (combining power) – in this case 1 for sodium. For non-metals the number of electrons gained by each atom is its valency and this is equal to 8 minus its group number. So for chlorine its valency is 1, i.e. 8 – 7.

Ionic compounds will conduct electricity when molten or dissolved in water since they dissociate into ions. They are called electrolytes, the electrical current is carried by the ions present. Electrolytes are very important in the body for the conduction of nerve impulses and muscle contraction as well as maintaining body fluid balance.

Some electrolytes are single ions such as the sodium ion (Na$^+$) and the chloride ion (Cl$^-$) however some ions are a collection of atoms, e.g. bicarbonate (HCO$_3^-$). These are known as polyatomic ions. Even though the bicarbonate ion (HCO$_3^-$) contains three atoms it still behaves as a simple ion with a negative charge (Table 1.5).

Covalent bonds – sharing electrons to make a full outer shell

When two non-metal atoms react together they obtain a full outer shell by sharing electrons between them. The compound formed is called a molecule and the bond holding the atoms

Table 1.5 Functions of polyatomic ions in the body

Polyatomic ion	Function
Ammonium ion (NH_4^+)	Regulates the acidity of urine
Dihydrogen phosphate ($H_2PO_4^-$)	Regulates the acidity of urine
Monohydrogen phosphate (HPO_4^{2-})	Regulates the acidity of urine
Bicarbonate (HCO_3^-)	Regulates the acidity of blood
Phosphate (PO_4^{3-})	Part of bone. One of the units of adenosine triphosphate (ATP) – the body's energy source

Exercise 1.2

Draw electron diagrams to show the formation of magnesium chloride ($MgCl_2$).

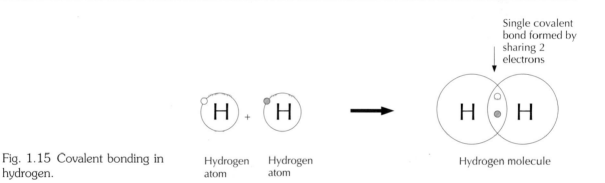

Single covalent bond formed by sharing 2 electrons

Hydrogen atom   Hydrogen atom

Hydrogen molecule

Fig. 1.15 Covalent bonding in hydrogen.

together in the molecule is a covalent bond. Molecules come in all shapes and sizes. They can contain just two atoms, such as hydrogen or they can contain millions of atoms as in DNA (deoxyribonucleic acid), or they can fall somewhere between the two (Table 1.6).

The formation of covalent bonds can be illustrated by looking at some simple molecules.

Hydrogen

A hydrogen atom has one electron in its outer shell and obtains a full shell by sharing this electron with another hydrogen atom (Fig. 1.15). A single covalent bond is represented by a line, so

the hydrogen molecule can be written as either H–H or H_2.

Chlorine

Chlorine has seven electrons in its outer shell and obtains a full shell by sharing one of these electrons with another chlorine atom (Fig. 1.16). A single covalent bond is represented by a line, so the chlorine molecule can be written as either Cl–Cl or Cl_2.

Since only the electrons in the outer shell react, only this shell is shown for simplicity. When covalent bonds are broken free radicals may be formed. A free radical is represented

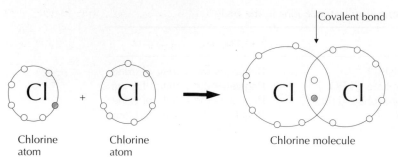

Chlorine atom + Chlorine atom → Chlorine molecule

Covalent bond

Fig. 1.16 Covalent bond in chlorine.

Table 1.6 Molecules

Molecule	Formula	Shape	Molecular mass
Hydrogen	H_2	Linear H–H	2 g
Water	H_2O	Bent or V shape	18 g
Ammonia	NH_3	Pyramidal	17 g
Glucose	$C_6H_{12}O_6$	Ring	180 g
Amino acid	alanine	Tetrahedral	89 g
DNA	deoxyribonucleic acid	Double helix	very large

by a dot, e.g. chlorine free radical, Cl•. Free radicals are very reactive as they have an unpaired electron. In the body they cause a wide range of reactions from age spots to wrinkles, kidney and liver disease and cancer. Free radicals cause irreversible damage to biological

---

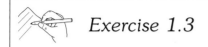

Exercise 1.3

Draw an electron diagram for the oxygen molecule (O_2).
How many covalent bonds does it have?

Table 1.7 Summary of differences between covalent and ionic bonds

Ionic	Covalent
Metal bonded to a non-metal	Non-metal bonded to a non-metal
Electron transfer	Sharing of electrons
Ions formed – force of attraction between ions holds compound together	No ions formed
Solids at room temp, with high melting and boiling points	Solids, liquids or gases with low melting points and boiling points
When molten or dissolved in water, conduct electricity – electrolytes	Do not conduct electricity – non-electrolytes
Mostly soluble in water	Mostly insoluble in water

---

molecules such as proteins and nucleic acids. The body produces substances called antioxidants to counteract the effect of these free radicals. Antioxidants work by donating an electron to the free radical thereby stabilising it. Nutrients such as vitamins A, C and E and the minerals selenium and zinc also function as antioxidants.

The differences between ionic and covalent bonds are summarised in Table 1.7.

Polar and non-polar covalent molecules

Electronegative atoms such as oxygen and nitrogen pull the electrons in the covalent bond towards themselves, resulting in unequal sharing of the bonded electrons (Fig. 1.17). The V-shaped water molecule, H_2O is described as polar. The oxygen atom becomes partially negatively charged, due to excess electrons and this is shown by the δ^-ve. The hydrogen becomes partially positive, shown by δ^+ve, due to the oxygen having the greater share of the bonded electrons. Polar molecules are attracted to other polar molecules and charged particles.

Molecules such as carbon dioxide and methane (natural gas) are non-polar (Fig. 1.18). In carbon dioxide the electron pulling power of one oxygen atom is cancelled out by that of the other oxygen atom.

The mole

A dozen, a score and a gross are all words that make us think of a number.

*This separation of charge is called a **dipole***

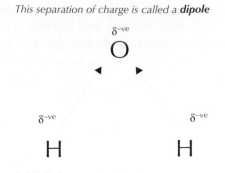

Fig. 1.17 Polar covalent molecule.

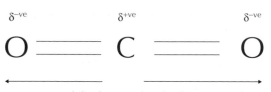

equal dipoles cancel each other out exactly

Fig. 1.18 Non-polar molecules.

If you ask a shopkeeper for a dozen eggs he will give you 12 eggs, if you ask him for a dozen doughnuts he will give you 12 doughnuts. So the word dozen always means 12 whatever you are buying. A score is always 20 and a gross is always 144.

Chemists deal with atoms. Atoms are very small particles and a dozen atoms would only have a tiny mass. Chemists therefore use the word 'mole' to describe a specific number. The mole is the amount of substance which contains 6.02×10^{23} particles (atoms, ions or molecules). The symbol for the mole unit is 'mol'. The number 6×10^{23} is called Avogadro's constant (old name Avogadro's number). Avogadro's constant is represented by the symbol N_A and is defined as the number of atoms in exactly 12 g of the carbon-12 isotope.

So think of the mole as an amount which contains a fixed number, a very large number but still a number, in the same way that a dozen always means 12 or a gross means 144.

One mole of any element will be its relative atomic mass expressed in grams. (See p. 227). Therefore for sodium:

1   mole of sodium atoms will have a mass of 23 g and contain 6×10^{23} atoms.

½   mole of sodium atoms will have a mass of ½ (23 g) and contain ½ (6×10^{23}) atoms.

2   moles of sodium atoms will have a mass of 2 (23 g) and contain 2 (6×10^{23}) atoms.

The mass of one mole of substance is called the molar mass. The symbol for molar mass is M and its units are normally grams per mole (g/mol or gmol^{-1}). Since the molar mass of an element is the mass per mole, it follows that the molar mass of carbon is 12.0 g/mol

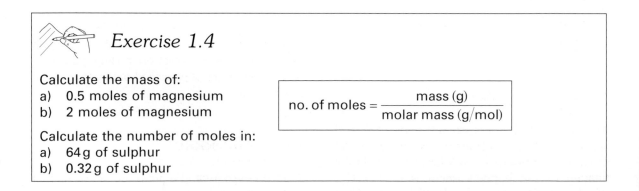

Exercise 1.4

Calculate the mass of:
a)   0.5 moles of magnesium
b)   2 moles of magnesium

Calculate the number of moles in:
a)   64 g of sulphur
b)   0.32 g of sulphur

$$\text{no. of moles} = \frac{\text{mass (g)}}{\text{molar mass (g/mol)}}$$

and that one mole of carbon has a mass of 12.0 g.

The term molar mass applies to all particles – atoms, molecules and ions. To avoid confusion the type of particle must be specified,

e.g.   1 mole of chlorine atoms have a mass of 35.5 g (molar mass 35.5 g/mol),
1 mole of chlorine molecules have a mass of 71.0 g (molar mass 71.0 g/mol).

Relative formula mass

The relative formula mass of a compound is calculated by adding all the relative atomic masses of the individual atoms together. The relative atomic masses of the individual atoms are found in the periodic table (see p. 227).

So the relative formula mass of sodium bicarbonate is calculated as follows:

Sodium bicarbonate, $NaHCO_3$:

$$23 \ + \ 1 \ + \ 12 \ + \ (16 \times 3) = 84$$
$$\uparrow \quad \uparrow \quad \uparrow \qquad \uparrow$$
$$Na \quad H \quad C \qquad O$$

The mass of one mole of sodium bicarbonate is its relative formula mass expressed in grams, i.e. 84 g.

For molecules the term relative molecular mass is used, so the relative molecular mass of glucose is calculated as follows:

Glucose, $C_6H_{12}O_6$:

$$(12 \times 6) + (1 \times 12) + (16 \times 6) = 180$$
$$\uparrow \qquad\quad \uparrow \qquad\qquad \uparrow$$
$$C \qquad\quad H \qquad\qquad O$$

The mass of one mole of glucose is its relative molecular mass expressed in grams, i.e. 180 g. Nurses need to be familiar with the concept of the mole since laboratory test results for blood, electrolytes, urea and glucose are expressed in moles.

Summary

- Atoms are the smallest particles, they are made up of protons, neutrons and electrons
- All known elements are found in the periodic table. They can be divided into metals and non-metals
- Isotopes are atoms of the same element which have the same atomic number but a different mass number, i.e. a different number of neutrons
- Compounds are formed when atoms are joined by chemical bonds
- Ionic bonds are formed by electron transfer between a metal and a non-metal
- Covalent bonds are formed by electron sharing between two non-metals
- Ions are charged atoms, positive ions are cations and negative ions anions
- A free radical is a species that has an unpaired electron
- A mole is made up of 6×10^{23} particles
- One mole of any atom will be its relative atomic mass expressed in grams.

Review questions

1.1.   Chromium-51 is used for red blood cell analysis, calculate the number of electrons, protons and neutrons it has?

$$^{51}_{24}Cr$$

1.2.   Work out the mass of one mole of:
(a)   carbon dioxide, CO_2
(b)   methane, CH_4
(c)   sucrose, $C_{12}H_{22}O_{11}$

1.3.   Predict the type of bonding (ionic or covalent) found in the following compounds:
(a)   water
(b)   carbon dioxide
(c)   potassium chloride
(d)   haemoglobin.

1.4.   Why are burns from steam potentially more dangerous than burns from hot water?

1.5.   Doctors prescribe ferrous sulphate tablets for anaemia, what metal do these tablets contain?

Further reading

Watson, R. (ed) (1999). *Essential Science for Nursing Students*. Baillière Tindall, London.

Sackheim, G.I. & Lechman, D.D. (1998). *Chemistry for the Health Sciences* (8th edn). Prentice Hall, London.

Cree, L. & Rischmiller, S. (1995). *Science in Nursing* (3rd edn). Baillière Tindall, London.

Chapter Two
WATER AND ELECTROLYTE BALANCE

Learning objectives

By the end of this chapter the reader will be able to:
- Describe the structure of the water molecule
- Explain how hydrogen bonds are formed
- Explain the terms surface tension, capillarity and meniscus
- Explain why some substances dissolve in water
- Distinguish between solvent, solute, solutions, colloids and suspensions
- List the units of concentration
- Define the terms diffusion, osmosis and filtration
- Explain the terms osmotic pressure, osmole and tonicity
- Describe what is meant by the terms electrolyte and non-electrolyte
- List and distinguish between the main fluid compartments in the body
- Describe water regulation in the body
- Briefly describe dialysis.

Introduction

The need to take in and eliminate water in order to maintain the water balance of the body is obvious. Have you ever been thirsty, or ever needed to go to the toilet desperately?

Imagine a shipwrecked sailor afloat in a lifeboat in the middle of the ocean. He has no fresh water to drink but is surrounded by water. Why can he not drink sea water to quench his thirst? By the end of this chapter you will be able to answer this question and explain the importance of water and electrolytes in the body.

Bonding in water

Water covers two-thirds of the earth's surface and is the most abundant molecule in your body. Water (H_2O) is a covalent polar molecule (Fig. 2.1).

The oxygen atom in water has 2 non-bonded pairs of electrons and 2 bonded pairs of electrons. The electron pairs try to get as far away from each other as possible. Water is bent or V-shaped due to the repulsion between these electron pairs (Fig. 2.2).

Hydrogen bonding

Hydrogen bonds are formed when a hydrogen atom forms a bridge between two electronegative atoms such as oxygen or nitrogen (Fig. 2.3). In water, the partially positive hydrogen atom of one water molecule is attracted to the partially negative oxygen atom of another water molecule. Therefore, water molecules attract each other via these hydrogen bonds. Hydrogen bonds are also found in a large

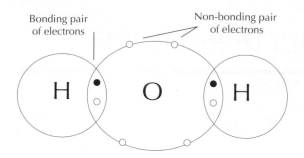

Fig. 2.1 Bonding in water.

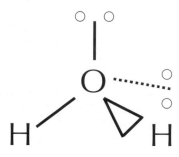

Fig. 2.2 The V-shape of water.

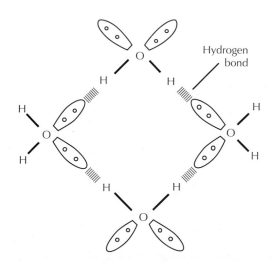

Fig. 2.3 Hydrogen bonding in water.

number of biological molecules, e.g. proteins, and are responsible for their shape. Hydrogen bonds are much weaker than ionic or covalent bonds.

Surface tension

Surface tensions vary between liquids. Water has a high surface tension and is a poor wetting agent because it forms droplets, e.g. raindrops on a windscreen. The surface of water forms a 'film' or 'skin', which can be strong enough for some insects, such as a pondskater, to walk on.

Cohesion is the force of attraction between 'like' molecules. In the middle of a container of water all the molecules experience the same cohesive forces. Molecules at the surface of the water do not experience these forces. These molecules are therefore 'drawn' into the body of the liquid, minimising the surface area and forming a drop (Fig. 2.4).

Alcohol has a lower surface tension than water. For this reason alcohol solutions are frequently used as antiseptics in hospitals since they wet the surface of the skin or equipment to be cleaned more thoroughly than water. Alcohol also evaporates faster than water, leaving the surface dry. Alcohol solutions are flammable and care should be taken when using these solutions.

Surface tensions of liquids can be changed by the addition of 'wetting agents' – surfactant (**surf**ace **act**ive **a**gent). You use surfactants without thinking, to lower the surface tension of water when you add detergent to wash your clothes, or use soap to wash your hands. A phospholipid surfactant is also found in the alveoli of the lungs, this reduces the surface tension of the fluid that lines the alveoli. In premature babies, one of the major problems can be a condition called 'neonatal respiratory distress syndrome' (RDS). Because of the immaturity of the baby's lungs, there is insufficient surfactant and the alveoli may collapse. This can also occur in full-term babies. Administration of steroid therapy to the mother before birth helps the lungs of the fetus to mature. Synthetic surfactants can also be injected into the lungs of the newborn.

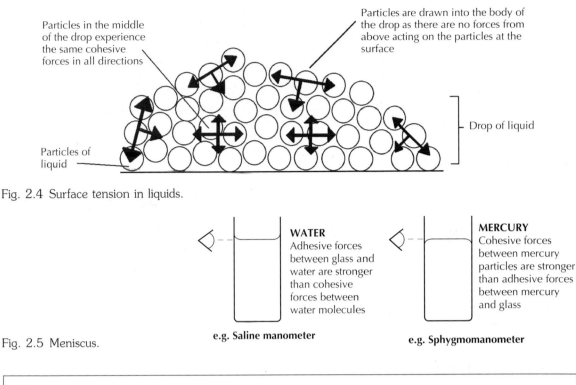

Particles in the middle of the drop experience the same cohesive forces in all directions

Particles are drawn into the body of the drop as there are no forces from above acting on the particles at the surface

Drop of liquid

Particles of liquid

Fig. 2.4 Surface tension in liquids.

Fig. 2.5 Meniscus.

WATER
Adhesive forces between glass and water are stronger than cohesive forces between water molecules

e.g. Saline manometer

MERCURY
Cohesive forces between mercury particles are stronger than adhesive forces between mercury and glass

e.g. Sphygmomanometer

✂ Activity

Fill a bowl with water. Sprinkle a teaspoon of flour onto the surface. Add one drop of washing-up liquid. Observe what happens to the surface tension of the water.

Meniscus

Adhesion is the forces of attraction between 'unlike' molecules. Forces of cohesion and adhesion give rise to the formation of a meniscus at the surface of liquids (Fig. 2.5).

Mercury has a convex meniscus since the cohesive forces are stronger than the adhesive forces. Water has a concave meniscus since the adhesive forces are greater than the cohesive forces.

Capillarity

Capillarity is the tendency of liquids to 'crawl' up the sides of tubes due to forces of adhesion (Fig. 2.6). Absorbent gauze and wick-type surgical drains all depend on capillarity to work. More importantly, normal blood pressure would be insufficient to move blood in capillaries without the effect of capillary action.

Water as a solvent

A solution consists of a solute and a solvent. The solvent is the substance that does the dissolving and the solute is the substance that is dissolved, e.g. in saline solution the solvent is water and the solute is sodium chloride (table salt).

Solute + Solvent = Solution

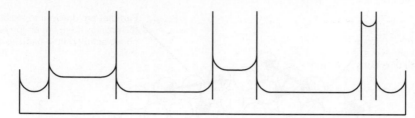

The narrower the tube, the greater the effect of capillarity and the higher the liquid travels up the tube

Fig. 2.6 The effect of capillarity.

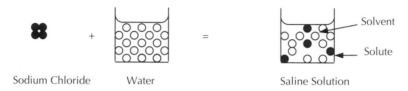

Sodium Chloride   Water   Saline Solution

Fig. 2.7 Solutions.

When sodium chloride dissolves in water, its particles spread out among the water particles (Fig. 2.7). The separate particles are too small to be seen and the solution looks 'clear'. These particles are so small they can pass through filter papers and cell membranes.

When water is the solvent, the solution is called an aqueous solution. Saturated solutions are solutions that can dissolve no more solid at a given temperature. As the temperature is increased, more solid will dissolve. An unsaturated solution is one that can dissolve more solid.

Water is an excellent solvent because of its structure – it is small and V-shaped. As a simple rule 'like dissolves like'. Water being a polar molecule will dissolve polar and ionic compounds. It dissolves these compounds because it can interact with them. When an ionic compound such as sodium chloride dissolves in water its ions separate. The positive ends of the water molecule are attracted to the negative ions (Cl^-) and the negative ends of the water molecule are attracted to the positive ions (Na^+). The attachment of solvent molecules to ions is

known as solvation or in the specific case of water hydration (Fig. 2.8). Polar, covalent compounds, e.g. alcohol and glucose contain –OH groups and dissolve in water since they are able to form hydrogen bonds with it. Substances that dissolve in water are called hydrophilic (water loving).

Non-polar covalent molecules, e.g. waxes, fats and steroids do not dissolve in water since water cannot interact with them. They are called hydrophobic (water hating) or lipophilic (fat loving). Non-polar compounds are soluble in non-polar solvents, e.g. hydrocarbons such as petrol and hexane.

To enter the body drugs need to be soluble. Non-polar drugs are fat soluble and can dissolve readily through the cell membranes so they can be administered as skin patches, pessaries or suppositories. Polar drugs are water soluble and can be administered orally or by intravenous (into the vein) injections since they are soluble in blood and body fluids.

There is also a link between solubility and how long a drug stays in the body (retention time). The more soluble a drug is in water

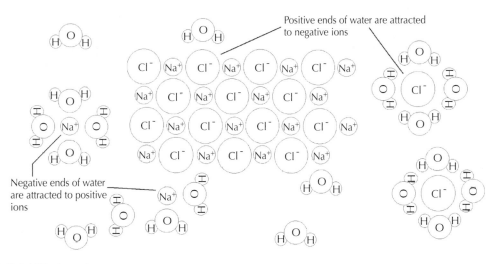

Fig. 2.8 Solubility in water.

the faster it is transported to the liver to be broken down and excreted in the urine so the shorter the retention time. Non-polar drugs tend to pass into cell membranes and fatty tissue and have a longer retention time however, they might not be soluble enough in blood to be effective. A balance can be struck between the two extremes and some drugs have polar and non-polar regions, e.g. the local anaesthetic lignocaine is transported in the body in water due to its polar region but it can also cross cell membranes due to its non-polar region.

Suspensions

In a suspension, solid particles do not separate fully. They clump together and are dispersed in the solvent but not dissolved (Fig. 2.9). The particles of a suspension cannot pass through filter papers or cell membranes. Blood is a suspension, the blood cells being suspended in a liquid called plasma. Constant movement of the blood keeps the erythrocytes (red blood cells) evenly distributed. Factors such as septicaemia, menstruation, inflammatory conditions and pregnancy can increase the erythrocyte sedimentation rate (ESR). As a result, erythrocytes can clump together. Clinically the erythrocyte sedimentation rate is measured to judge the progress of a disease.

A large number of medicines are suspensions – calamine lotion, Calpol®, penicillin, milk of magnesia. If a suspension is left to stand, the solid particles will separate out, therefore it is important to shake the medicine bottle before use, otherwise the incorrect dosage of medicine will be given.

Colloids

Colloidal particles are larger than those in a solution, but smaller than those in a suspension. Particle size is measured in nanometres (nm) (1 nm is 0.000 000 001 m). Colloidal particles range in size from 1 to 100 nm. Solution particles are much smaller, being less than 1 nm, suspension particles are much larger, being bigger than 100 nm. Colloids consist of clusters of particles or a very large molecule such as a protein, e.g. plasma. Because of their size colloidal particles can pass through filter papers, but are too big to pass through cell membranes. When the blood is filtered by the kidneys no proteins should pass through the glomerular endothelium membrane because they are too large,

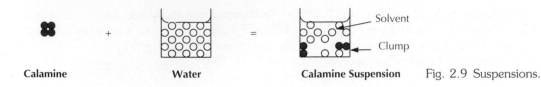

Calamine　+　Water　=　Calamine Suspension　　Fig. 2.9 Suspensions.

Solvent

Clump

Table 2.1 Different types of colloids

Type	Continuous Phase	Dispersed Phase	Clinical Examples	Everyday Example
sol	liquid	solid	plasma	paint
gel	solid	liquid	wound dressing – hydrogels	agar and gelatine
emulsion	liquid	liquid	formed in the digestion of fats by the action of bile salts	milk, hand cream and French dressing
aerosol	gas	liquid or solid	inhalation therapy; dry antibiotic spray	smoke and mist

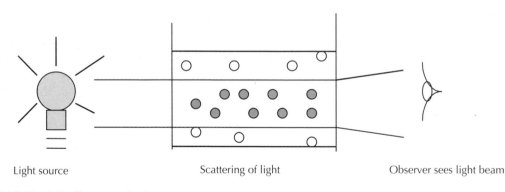

Light source　　　　Scattering of light　　　　Observer sees light beam

Fig. 2.10 Tyndall effect in colloids.

therefore no proteins should be found in the urine.

There are several different types of colloids made by dispersing one substance in another (Table 2.1). Colloids consist of at least two parts, for example in plasma the continuous phase is a watery liquid called serum and the dispersed phase is the proteins, albumin, globulin and fibrinogen found scattered or dispersed in the watery liquid.

Colloids can be distinguished from true solutions by shining light through the solution. The particles are large enough to scatter light, e.g.

car headlights in fog. This is known as the Tyndall effect (Fig. 2.10).

Crystalloid and colloid intravenous infusions

When fluids are given directly into a vein they are referred to as intravenous infusions (IV drip). Such infusions may be used to restore blood, fluid, electrolytes or administer drugs. Some intravenous fluids are colloidal suspensions. These include blood, albumin solution (95%

albumin) and plasma protein solution (85% albumin). All of these are derived from human donors. Synthetic plasma protein substitutes are also used, e.g. hetastarch, Hespan® or dextran, Gentran®. These are known as plasma expanders since they do not leak out of the blood vessels and maintain blood volume and increase blood pressure.

Crystalloid intravenous infusions include sodium chloride and glucose (dextrose) solutions. They are referred to as crystalloid because the solute can form crystals. As a nurse you must be aware that different intravenous infusions will be given depending on the need of the patient. However, before any intravenous infusion is given hospital protocols must be observed and these may include the following checks:

- expiry date and batch number
- packaging intact
- whether the fluid is clear (when appropriate)
- for the presence of any debris
- correct prescription for patient.

Concentrations

Concentration of a solution is the amount of solute dissolved in a given volume of solvent. In Fig. 2.11 there are three solutions of glucose in water. The amount of glucose dissolved in each varies but the same volume of water is used, 1 L. Each of the solutions has a different concentration.

Concentration can be expressed in several different forms; as a nurse you must be familiar with these different units.

Weight by weight (w/w)

Creams and ointments are usually expressed in w/w, e.g. hydrocortisone is 2.5% w/w and contains 2.5 g of hydrocortisone in 100 g of soft paraffin.

Volume by volume (v/v)

A 10% aqueous solution of alcohol contains 10 ml of alcohol made up to 100 ml with water, e.g. the inhalation preparation menthol and eucalyptus is 10% v/v.

Weight by volume (w/v)

A 10% aqueous solution of sodium chloride contains 10 g of sodium chloride made up to 100 mL with water. The two most common intravenous infusions are normal saline which is 0.9% w/v (i.e. 0.9 g of sodium chloride made up to 100 mL with water) and dextrose (glucose) which is 5% w/v (i.e. 5 g of glucose made up to 100 mL with water).

Weight by volume (mg/mL)

Another way of expressing w/v is mg/mL. The concentration of paracetamol in Calpol® is

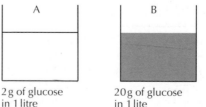

A	B	C
2 g of glucose in 1 litre of water. This is a **dilute** solution compared with B and C.	20 g of glucose in 1 lite of water. This solution is more **concentrated** than solution A.	200 g of glucose in 1 lite of water. This solution is more **concentrated** than solutions A and B.

Fig. 2.11 Concentrations of solutions.

expressed as 120 mg/5 mL. It is important to use the measuring spoon provided with the medicine. The volume 5 mL comes from the fact that most teaspoons are roughly 5 mL, so in an emergency a teaspoon could be used to administer the medicine.

Molarity

Molarity is the Système International (SI) unit of concentration. Molarity is the number of moles of solute per litre of solvent. The units of molarity are mol/L or molL^{-1}. Therefore 1 mole of any substance dissolved in 1 L of solvent has a concentration of 1.0 mol/L. (This is a 'molar' solution.) The concentrations of substances in the body, such as hormones and electrolytes, are usually very small, therefore millimoles per litre (mmol/L) are used instead (Table 2.2). A millimole is 1/1000 of a mole, i.e. 0.001 mol/L is the same as 1 mmol/L

$$\text{Concentration (mol/L)} = \frac{\text{number of moles}}{\text{volume of solution (L)}}$$

Read Chapter 1 to remind yourself that a mole of substance is its relative molecular mass in grams.

Example

Beaker A (Fig. 2.11) contains 2 g of glucose, dissolved in 1 L of water.

One mole of glucose = 180 g

$$\begin{aligned}\text{number of moles} \\ \text{of glucose}\end{aligned} = \frac{\text{Mass of glucose}}{\text{Molar mass}} = \frac{2}{180}$$

$$= 0.011 \text{ mol}$$

$$\text{Concentration of glucose} = \frac{0.011 \text{ mol}}{1 \text{ L}}$$

$$= 0.011 \text{ mol/L}$$

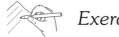

Exercise 2.1

Calculate the concentration of the glucose solutions in beakers B & C in Fig. 2.11.

Other units of concentration

Milliequivalent per litre (mEq/L)

This is a very old unit, but is still used in North America. The milliequivalent takes into account the charges carried by particles.

As you can see in Table 2.2, for ions with a single charge, molarity and milliequivalent have the same value. If the ion has a charge of 2, then the value of the milliequivalent is twice that of its molarity.

Table 2.2 Plasma electrolyte values

Electrolyte	SI Unit (mmol/L)	Older unit (mEq/L)
Bicarbonate HCO_3^-	21–30	21–30
Calcium Ca^{2+}	2.1–2.7	4.2–5.4
Chloride Cl^-	98–108	98–108
Magnesium Mg^{2+}	0.75–1.25	1.5–2.5
Potassium K^+	3.5–5.2	3.5–5.2
Sodium Na^+	135–146	135–146

■ ■ *Diffusion and osmosis*

Substances such as electrolytes, gases and nutrients need to move about the body. They can do this by passive or active transport systems.

■ *Passive transport*

Particles move by virtue of the kinetic energy they possess. This is sufficient to allow them to cross cell membranes. No additional energy is required.

■ *Active transport*

Additional energy in the form of adenosine triphosphate (ATP) is required, which is provided by the cell. Without this extra energy, movement would not be achieved.

Diffusion and osmosis are both examples of passive transport. Exocytosis and endocytosis are examples of active transport.

■ *Diffusion*

Diffusion is defined as the movement of particles (molecules, ions and atoms) from an area of high concentration to an area of low concentration. This is said to be 'down a concentration gradient' (Fig. 2.12).

Many substances diffuse in the body – fat soluble substances, small ions and gases. Diffusion is fast over short distances but is very slow over large distances, this is probably why cells are so small. Diffusion is also faster in gases than in liquids.

■ *Diffusion across a membrane*

A membrane is a barrier, which allows certain particles to pass through, but not others. Living cell membranes are called selectively permeable membranes, since they have the capacity to select which particles pass through. Non-living membranes (e.g. dialysis tubing) are called semipermeable membranes, since they only separate large particles from small particles.

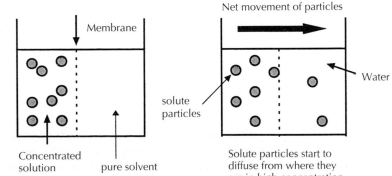
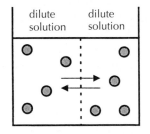

Fig. 2.12 Diffusion.

Factors that affect the rate of diffusion include:

Surface area	Size of particle	Thickness of membrane
Concentration	Temperature	Distance
Charge	Pressure	particle has to move

A large number of conditions are associated with poor diffusion of gases:

- Emphysema – increases the size of the alveoli hence decreasing the surface area of the lungs leading to poor gas exchange
- Pulmonary fibrosis – increases the thickness of the alveoli membranes decreasing gas exchange
- Oedema – swollen waterlogged tissue tends to be more vulnerable to damage and slower to heal since the water in the tissue is an increased barrier to the diffusion of oxygen and nutrients.

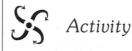 *Activity*

a) In a closed room, spray some perfume into the air. Note how quickly you can smell the odour of the perfume. Leave the room for a few minutes and re-enter. Notice how much the odour of the perfume now fills the room.
b) Take a glass of water and drop some ink onto the surface of the water. Note how the ink particles slowly diffuse through the water. Compare this with how quickly the perfume particles spread through the air. Stir the water with a spoon and notice what happens.

Facilitated diffusion

Facilitated diffusion moves large fat (lipid) insoluble molecules such as glucose across the cell membrane (Fig. 2.13). The substance to be transported is bound to a protein carrier which is specific to that substance. This is still diffusion down a concentration gradient. Facilitated diffusion is limited by the number of protein carriers available and when all the carriers are busy saturation is reached – this is referred to as the threshold or transport maximum. The hormone insulin is involved in glucose transport and affects the rate at which glucose is transported into the cell.

Osmosis

Osmosis is the diffusion of a solvent across a membrane. In living things the solvent is always water. The human body contains a high percentage of water and osmosis is continually

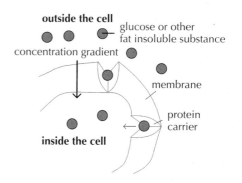

Fig. 2.13 Facilitated diffusion.

moving water in and out of cells. Osmotic imbalances in the body can result in cells swelling and shrinking, dehydration and diarrhoea, and are one of the causes of oedema.

Osmosis is defined as the movement of water (solvent) across a selectively permeable membrane, from an area of high water (solvent) concentration to an area of low water (solvent) concentration (Fig. 2.14).

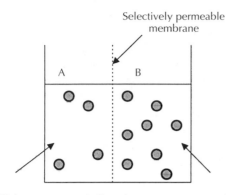

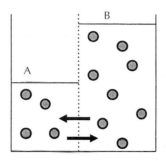

High water concentration   Low water concentration

Net movement of water

Solute particles are too big
to pass through the
selectively permeable membrane.
Water molecules pass through
by osmosis from A to B.

No net movement of water at equilibrium

Water has moved across the
selectively permeable membrane
from A to B, until the concentrations
of the two solutions are equal at
equilibrium. This is a dynamic process
with water molecules passing in both
directions across the membrane.

Fig. 2.14 Osmosis.

Osmotic pressure

Osmotic pressure of a solution is the pressure needed to prevent the movement of water by osmosis. The greater the difference in concentration between the two solutions on either side of the selectively permeable membrane the greater the osmotic pressure needed to stop the movement of water by osmosis. Osmotic pressure is often referred to as the 'osmotic pull' since it appears to pull water through the membrane.

The osmotic pressure of a solution depends on the *number*, not the type, of particles dissolved in solution (Fig. 2.15). Electrolytes such as sodium chloride generate a larger osmotic pressure than non-electrolytes since they dissociate into ions in solution. Non-electrolytes such as glucose remain intact.

$$Na\,Cl \rightarrow Na^+ + Cl^-\ \text{two particles}$$
$$C_6H_{12}O_6 \rightarrow \text{one particle}$$

Osmolarity and osmolality

The concentration of a solute in terms of its number of particles is expressed by a unit called the osmole.

The concentration of a solution in osmoles is given in two ways:

(a) Osmolarity (units osmol/L)

osmolarity = molarity × number of
             dissociated solute particles:

the osmolarity of 1 mol/L sodium chloride solution is:

1 (number of moles) × 2 (number of
    particles) = 2 osmol/L

The osmolarity of 1 mol/L glucose solution is:

$1 \times 1 = 1\,\text{osmol/L}$

Since the concentrations of substances in the body are very low milliosmoles (mosmol/L) are used.

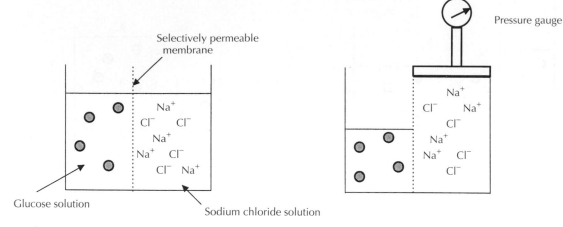

Fig. 2.15 Effect of electrolytes on osmosis.

A solution with a greater osmolarity than another is referred to as being 'hyperosmotic'. One with a lower osmolarity, compared to another, is referred to as 'hypo-osmotic'. Two solutions that have the same osmolarity are referred to as 'iso-osmotic'.

(b) Osmolality (units osmol/kg)
A molal solution is one in which 1 mole of solute is contained in 1 kg of solvent.

$$\text{Osmolality} = \text{molality} \times \text{number of ions in solution}$$

In the body the solvent is always water and as 1 litre of water weighs almost exactly 1 kg therefore the two units (osmolarity and osmolality) are virtually identical.

Tonicity of cells

Tonicity is the ability of a solution to vary the size and shape of cells by changing the amount of water in the cell (Fig. 2.16).

Normal saline (0.9% w/v sodium chloride solution) and 5% w/v glucose (dextrose) solution are both isotonic with plasma and are commonly used for intravenous infusions. Neither of these two solutions are plasma, but they do have the same concentrations of particles. Sea water is hypertonic relative to body fluids having a sodium chloride concentration of 1 mol/L. Drinking sea water would therefore cause water to leave the cells by osmosis, resulting in dehydration. Most of the fluids that you drink, e.g. tea or fruit juice, are hypotonic relative to your body fluids.

Activity

Peel a potato and cut it in half. Dig out a cavity in one half of the potato. Half fill the cavity with a concentrated salt solution. Place the potato 'cup' in a dish of water. Mark the level of the salt solution, by sticking a pin in the potato. Note what happens to the level of the salt solution after 30 min. Explain.

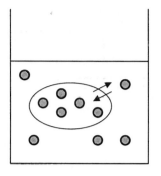

Isotonic solution

In an isotonic solution has the same concentration of dissolved substances either side of membrane. Water moves in and out of the cell, but there is no net movement of water – retains shape.

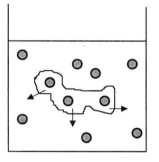

Hypertonic solution

In a hypertonic solution the solute concentration is higher outside the cell than inside. Water will move out of the cell into the solution, by osmosis, causing the cell to shrink – this is *crenation*.

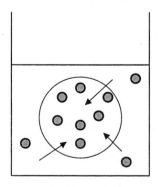

Hypotonic solution

In a hypotonic solution the solute concentration is lower outside the cell than inside. Water will move into the cell from the solution by osmosis, causing the cell to swell and burst – this is *haemolysis*.

Fig. 2.16 Effect of tonicity on the red blood cell.

Filtration

Filtration occurs in the capillaries where liquid is forced out into the interstitial spaces by hydrostatic pressure (blood pressure) and in the kidneys where it is the start of urine formation. Filtration is the process by which water and solutes are forced through a membrane by pressure, large particles are left behind or removed, e.g. proteins and blood cells (Fig. 2.17). Filtration occurs due to a difference in pressure on either side of the membrane – a pressure gradient. The pressure used for filtration in the body is blood pressure.

Electrolyte balance

Electrolytes when dissolved in water dissociate into ions. The most important electrolytes in the body are the cations sodium (Na^+), potassium (K^+), magnesium (Mg^{2+}), calcium (Ca^{2+}), hydrogen (H^+), and the anions bicarbonate (HCO_3^-), chloride (Cl^-), phosphate (PO_4^{3-}) and sulphate (SO_4^{2-}). H^+ ion concentration controls pH (see Chapter 3) the other ions control the electrolyte balance.

Non-electrolytes are covalently bonded compounds, e.g. glucose, lipids and urea. They do not dissociate into ions in solution and do not conduct electricity. Doctors frequently request U&E and GLC on laboratory request cards, this abbreviation stands for urea, electrolytes and glucose.

Disturbances in electrolyte concentrations are relatively common and the terms used to describe them are made up of three parts (Fig. 2.18).

The concentrations of electrolytes in the body are maintained within narrow ranges (Table 2.2 and Fig. 2.21). The body can excrete electrolytes in the urine via the kidneys if they are in excess or reabsorb them if the concentration

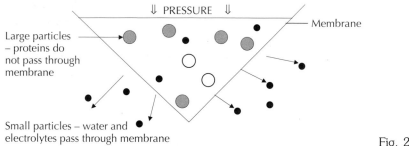
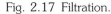

Large particles – proteins do not pass through membrane

Membrane

Small particles – water and electrolytes pass through membrane

Fig. 2.17 Filtration.

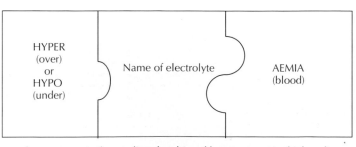

HYPER (over) or HYPO (under)

Name of electrolyte

AEMIA (blood)

e.g. hyponatraemia (low sodium levels) and hypernatraemia (high sodium levels) – also hypokalaemia (low potassium levels) and hyperkalaemia (high potassium levels).

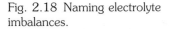

Fig. 2.18 Naming electrolyte imbalances.

of electrolytes falls below normal. Electrolytes are also lost through sweat and the gastrointestinal tract as faeces. Hormones (antidiuretic, parathyroid, adrenal hormones and atrial natriuretic peptide) also play a major part in water and electrolyte balance.

Water in the body

Water cannot be stored in the body yet 60% of total body weight is water. Excessive vomiting or a long bout of diarrhoea can be life-threatening if the lost water and electrolytes are not replaced. This is even more the case with babies since they have a higher water content (70%). A patient suffering third degree burns may die not from his burns but from the loss of water.

The percentage of water in the body depends on age, sex and the amount of fat. Fat tissue (adipose tissue) contains less water than bone (Table 2.3).

There are two main fluid compartments in the body (Fig. 2.19):

(1) INTRACELLULAR FLUID COMPARTMENT (ICF) – fluid inside the cell
(2) EXTRACELLULAR FLUID COMPARTMENT (ECF) – fluid outside the cell

The ECF is sub-divided into two compartments:
a) plasma (intravascular) compartment
b) interstitial fluid (fluid between cells).

There are also specialised body fluids such as lymph, cerebrospinal fluid, humours of the eye and synovial fluid found in joints. Their compositions are very similar to interstitial fluid and they can be considered as part of it.

Fluid movement – formation of interstitial fluid

The movement of body fluids between compartments is regulated by osmotic and/or hydrostatic pressure (blood pressure). Exchanges between plasma and interstitial fluid occurs across capillary walls (Fig. 2.20).

Capillaries connect arterioles and venules. Therefore, along the length of a capillary the hydrostatic pressure will vary from 32 mm Hg at the arterial end to 12 mm Hg at the venous end. The hydrostatic pressure in capillaries tends to force fluid out of the capillaries. The osmotic pressure of the plasma proteins (oncotic pressure) *opposes* this flow. Albumin is the main plasma protein responsible for maintaining the osmotic pressure in plasma. The osmotic pres-

Table 2.3 Water as a percentage of bodyweight

Age	Newborn	1 year	20–39 year		40–60 year	
			Male	Female	Male	Female
% water	80	70	60	50	55	47

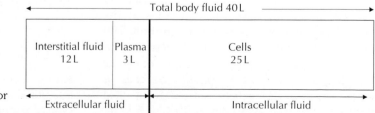

Fig. 2.19 Water in the body (values for 70 kg male).

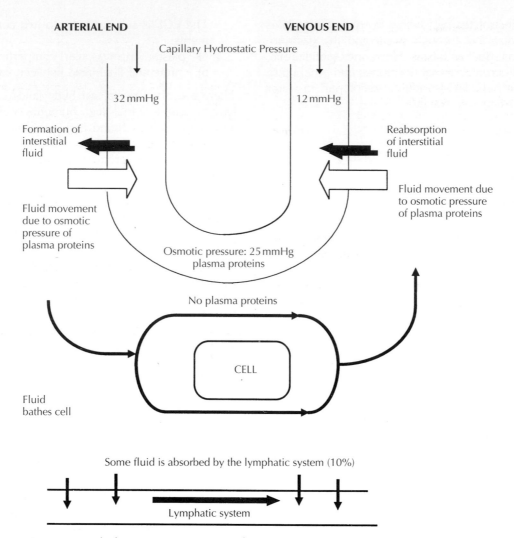

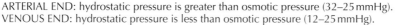

ARTERIAL END: hydrostatic pressure is greater than osmotic pressure (32–25 mmHg).
VENOUS END: hydrostatic pressure is less than osmotic pressure (12–25 mmHg).

Fig. 2.20 Summary of fluid movement.

sure due to the plasma proteins is relatively constant along the length of the capillary at 25 mmHg. Fluid leaves the capillaries at the arterial end and returns at the venous end. The pores in the capillary walls only allow small molecules to leave the capillaries and the interstitial fluid that bathes the cell contains no cells or large proteins. Approximately 20 L of fluid moves in this way every day – 90% of it is re-

absorbed at the venous end whilst 10% goes into the lymph system.

Oedema

An oedema is the excessive accumulation of interstitial fluid, which causes the tissue to swell. One of the characteristics of oedema is 'pitting'.

Table 2.4 Formation of oedema

Physiological mechanism	Example
Increased capillary hydrostatic pressure – causes increased fluid flow out of the capillary	Pregnancy, tight bandage or plaster, varicose veins. Excessive administration of intravenous infusions
Decrease in plasma protein osmotic pressure – decreases the reabsorption of fluid	Liver damage, burns, malnutrition (kwashiorkor) and starvation all lower blood proteins (hypoproteinaemia)
Increased permeability of capillary walls – causes an increased fluid flow out of the capillary	Inflammatory response or allergic reaction – due to the release of histamine
Decrease in lymphatic removal – decrease in the reabsorption of fluid into the lymphatic system	Surgical removal of the lymph nodes, infestation by the parasitic worm, filaria (elephantiasis), lymphoedema. Tumour in lymph ducts

If the skin of the oedema is pressed with a finger, a 'pit' appears and remains for approx. 30 s. There are many causes of oedema, but there are only four main physiological mechanisms for their formation (Table 2.4).

Exercise 2.2

Use Fig. 2.21 to answer the following questions:
1. Which is the most abundant cation in intracellular fluid?
2. Which is the most abundant cation in extracellular fluid?
3. Which is the most abundant anion in extracellular fluid?

Water balance

Under normal conditions the water intake each day is roughly equal to the water excreted (Fig. 2.22). Clinically, the best guide to changes in body water is alteration in bodyweight.

Dehydration occurs when water loss exceeds water intake over a period of time. As water is lost electrolytes are also lost; however, the loss of water is greater. Dehydration commonly occurs after severe burns, haemorrhage, or prolonged bouts of vomiting or diarrhoea. Excessive urine output as in diabetes (mellitus or insipidus) also results in dehydration. In the elderly or very young and with patients in hospitals, dehydration may result from the inability to obtain water themselves, so always check on a ward that the water jugs are full, regularly changed and in easy reach of the patient.

Hypertonic dehydration results from the loss of extracellular fluid. Water will leave the cell by osmosis to compensate for this loss. Cells begin to shrink and this is reflected in the tissues by sunken eyeballs, dry or 'cottony' mucous of the mouth and dry skin. If the dehydration becomes severe then the neurones in the brain will start to shrink causing confusion, convulsions and eventually death. So the shipwrecked sailor had better hurry up and get a drink!

Hypotonic hydration (water intoxication) results when the extracellular fluid (ECF) is diluted and may cause vomiting, muscular cramping and cerebral oedema. Low levels of sodium in the ECF result in hyponatraemia and

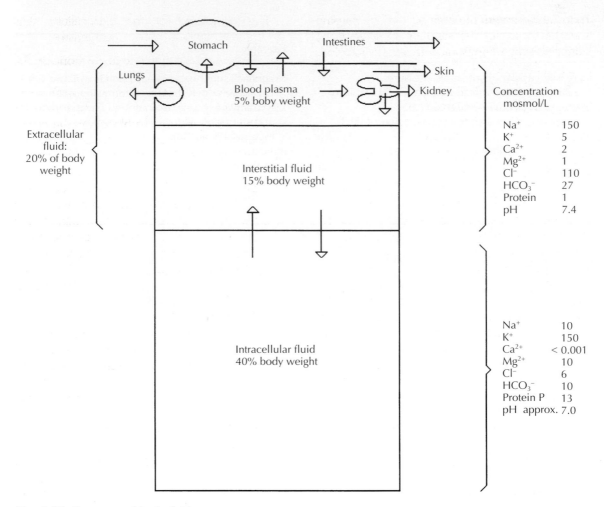

Fig. 2.21 Summary of body fluids.

(⇑ arrow indicates that intake and output can increase greatly).

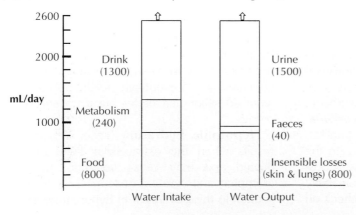

Fig. 2.22 Water balance in a young male.

more water enters the cells by osmosis causing the cell to swell. The situation is reversed by administering a hypotonic intravenous infusion.

Water regulation

Body fluids in a healthy adult are maintained within a narrow range (285–300 mosmol/L) despite large changes in sodium and water intake. Sodium, as the main extracellular cation, regulates the osmolarity of the extracellular fluid (ECF). Since intracellular and extracellular fluids are normally isotonic, sodium ions control the osmolarity of the whole body. Sodium ions also determine and regulate the volume of extracellular fluids – 'water follows sodium'. So even when the sodium concentration in the body changes, its concentration in the ECF remains constant due to changes in water volume.

Sodium intake is not regulated and in western diets we take in 10–15 g of sodium a day, we only need 1 g. Excess sodium in the diet can result in hypertension (high blood pressure). Sodium is lost by sweating and in faeces but the main organ responsible for the loss and regulation of sodium is the kidneys. Salt should not be added to babies' food, since their kidneys are too immature to cope.

The osmolarity of the extracellular fluid (blood) is controlled by two mechanisms:

(1) The release of antidiuretic hormone (ADH, alternative name vasopressin)

Within the hypothalamus of the brain there are cells (osmoreceptors) which monitor the osmolarity of the blood. As the osmolarity of the blood rises, these osmoreceptors signal the release of antidiuretic hormone from the posterior lobe of the pituitary gland located beneath the brain. ADH increases the retention of water and the production of urine with a high sodium concentration. A decrease in osmotic pressure causes a decrease in the secretion of ADH with increased loss of water by the kidney and an increase in urine output (diuresis) (Fig. 2.23).

(2) Thirst mechanisms

If the osmolarity of the blood rises the thirst centre in the hypothalamus is excited which motivates the person to drink. Thirst is quenched almost as soon as we start to drink, this prevents us from drinking too much and allows time for the water to be absorbed and osmotic equilibrium to be restored. The thirst receptors are not usually triggered until ADH is released, this is to ensure that all water drunk is retained by the kidneys (Fig. 2.23).

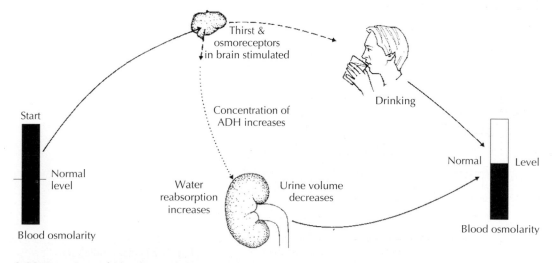

Fig. 2.23 Summary of blood osmolarity.

Dialysis

The kidneys are responsible for controlling the fluid and electrolyte balance in the body and the excretion of waste products e.g. urea. When renal failure occurs dialysis takes over the work done by the kidneys. Dialysis cannot totally replace lost renal function, the only way to do this is through a kidney transplant.

Dialysis is the movement of solutes through a semi-permeable membrane by diffusion down a concentration gradient. In haemodialysis, an artificial membrane enclosed within a dialyser is used. In peritoneal dialysis, the body's own peritoneum acts as the dialytic membrane. The peritoneum is a double-layered membrane that lines the interior of the abdominal cavity and surfaces of the abdominal organs.

Haemodialysis

In haemodialysis blood is withdrawn from the body and pumped through an 'artificial kidney' or dialyser and then back into the body (Fig. 2.24). The blood flows along one side of the semi-permeable membrane and a special fluid called the dialysate flows on the other side of the membrane. The dialysate is mostly water but may also contain substances such as glucose and bicarbonate.

Large molecules such as blood cells and proteins cannot pass through the dialyser membrane. However the membrane does allow the passage of small molecules, e.g. potassium ions, creatinine and urea by diffusion down their concentration gradients. Depending on their concentration small molecules can diffuse from the blood into the dialystate (urea, potassium and creatinine), or from the dialystate to the blood (glucose and bicarbonate). The dialysate is continually pumped and its flow is opposite to that of the blood (countercurrent) so that these concentration gradients are maintained.

A pressure gradient also exists over each side of the dialysis membrane and is described as the transmembrane pressure. This allows for the filtration of water and other solutes from the blood. Changing the pressure gradient allows more or less water to be removed from the blood as it moves through the dialyser. Dialysis is an ongoing treatment and is done on average three times a week, each session lasting 3–6 hours depending on the patient.

Peritoneal dialysis

The patient's own peritoneal membrane is the dialytic membrane. The dialysing solution is placed in the peritoneal cavity using an indwelling catheter and left to equilibrate for

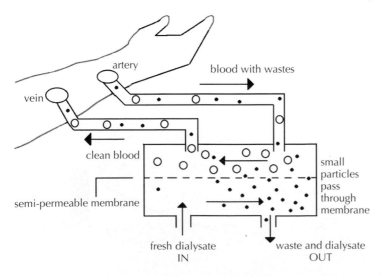

Fig. 2.24 Haemodialysis.

4–6 hours. The dialysate is then removed and replaced with more fresh dialysing fluid. Changing the concentration of glucose in the dialysate changes its osmolarity and this regulates the movement of water by osmosis from the blood to the dialysate. This process can be carried out by the patient in their own home. Peritonitis is a common complication of this treatment.

 Activity

A variety of dialysates are used for dialysis depending on the patients needs. Look at bags of dialysate in a renal unit and find out what they contain and why there is such a variety.

Summary

- Water is a polar covalent molecule and can form hydrogen bonds
- 'Like dissolves like' – so polar solvents dissolve polar compounds, non-polar solvents dissolve non-polar compounds
- A solution consists of a solute and a solvent
- Solutions, colloids and suspensions are formed depending on the size of the solute particles
- The concentration of a solution is the amount of solute dissolved in a given volume of solvent
- Diffusion is the movement of particles down a concentration gradient
- Osmosis is the movement of water across a selectively permeable membrane
- The number of particles of a solute in solution is given in terms of osmolarity or osmolality
- Sodium ions help to regulate the osmolarity of body fluids
- Water is regulated in the body by the thirst mechanism and the antidiuretic hormone (ADH)
- Dialysis uses filtration, diffusion and osmosis to clean the blood.

Review questions

2.1. Are the following solutions suspensions or colloids?
  a) lemonade   c) shampoo
  b) toothpaste   d) chicken soup

2.2. Using osmosis explain how the laxative Epsom salts ($MgSO_4$) works. What advice would you give a patient taking this laxative?

2.3. Why are salty snacks, such as peanuts and crisps always sold in pubs and bars? Explain the effect of these snacks on the body.

2.4. Explain the difference between:
  a) osmosis and diffusion
  b) molarity and osmolarity

2.5. Blisters occur when shoes rub the skin. What is the physiological mechanism for the formation of a blister?

Further reading

Smith, E.K.M. (1991). *Fluids and Electrolytes. A conceptual approach* (2nd edn). Churchill Livingstone, New York.

Marieb E.N. (2000). *Human Anatomy and Physiology* (5th edn). Benjamin Cummings, Redwood City, California.

Tortora, G.J. and Grabowska, S.P. (1999). *Principles of Anatomy and Physiology* (9th edn). John Wiley & Sons Ltd, Chichester.

Chapter Three
ACIDS AND BASES

Learning objectives

By the end of this chapter the reader will be able to:
- Define the terms acid and base
- Define the term neutralisation
- Distinguish between strong and weak acids and bases
- Explain the pH scale in terms of hydrogen ion concentration
- Describe the main buffering systems in the body and how they maintain pH
- Explain the terms metabolic acidosis/alkalosis and respiratory acidosis/alkalosis.

Introduction

Acids and bases are common everyday substances. Oven cleaners, washing soda and caustic soda are household bases. Vinegar, car battery acid and lemon juice are household acids. In dilute solutions these substances pose little danger. However, in concentrated solutions acids and bases can be dangerous and corrosive.

Acids and bases are also found in the body. In the body their levels need to be regulated continually. If acid levels are too high (acidosis) or base levels are too high (alkalosis) the patient can become very ill – or even die. Treatment of patients suffering from acidosis and alkalosis is based on the way acids and bases react together.

Acids

The property that all acids have in common is that in solution they dissociate to donate (give) hydrogen ions H^+. For example hydrochloric acid:

$$HCl_{(aq)} \rightarrow H^+_{(aq)} + Cl^-_{(aq)}$$
hydrochloric   hydrogen ion   chloride ion

An acid is therefore defined as a hydrogen ion donor. A hydrogen ion is also known as a proton. There are a number of other ways we might recognise or describe an acid:

- having a sour taste
- being corrosive – burning tissue
- turning blue litmus red
- reacting with a base to form salt and water – neutralisation
- having a pH less than 7.

Table 3.1 lists a few examples of common acids.

Activity

If you look at the labels of the following foods which acids can you find in them?

a) cola   b) squash   c) pickled onions   d) jam

Table 3.1 Some common acids

ACID	NOTES
Acetylsalicylic acid (aspirin)	Derived from salicin found in willow bark analgesic and antipyretic; helps prevent blood clotting
Citric acid	Found in citrus fruits – lemons, limes; formed in the body when glucose is oxidised to give energy – Krebs cycle
Carbonic acid	Found in fizzy drinks; formed when carbon dioxide dissolves in water and is involved in regulation of body pH
Lactic acid	Found in sour milk and yoghurt; formed as the end product during anaerobic respiration, especially in muscles
Hydrochloric acid	Found in the stomach where it is involved in the digestion of proteins and in decreasing the bacteria count from ingested food
Folic acid	Member of the vitamin B group, taken in the first 3 months of pregnancy for normal neural tube development preventing spina bifida; deficiency can cause megaloblastic anaemia

Bases

Bases are the chemical opposites of acids. Bases are hydrogen ion acceptors. If a base is soluble in water then it is called an alkali. All alkalis are bases but not all bases are alkalis.

Alkalis dissociate in water to give the hydroxide ion OH^-

$$NaOH_{(aq)} \rightarrow Na^+_{(aq)} + OH^-_{(aq)}$$
sodium hydroxide   sodium ion   hydroxide ion

This hydroxide ion can then accept hydrogen ions to form water.

$$OH^-_{(aq)} + H^+_{(aq)} \rightarrow H_2O_{(l)}$$
hydroxide ion   hydrogen ion   water

There are also a number of other ways we might recognise or describe a base:

- having a bitter metallic taste
- being corrosive – burning tissue
- turning red litmus blue
- reacting with an acid to form salt plus water – neutralisation
- having a pH value greater than 7.

Table 3.2 lists a few common bases.

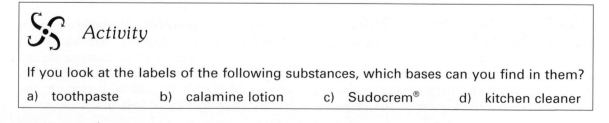

Activity

If you look at the labels of the following substances, which bases can you find in them?

a) toothpaste   b) calamine lotion   c) Sudocrem®   d) kitchen cleaner

Table 3.2 Some common bases

BASE	NOTES
Sodium hydroxide (caustic soda)	Strong cleaning agent especially for grease, e.g. oven cleaner
Magnesium hydroxide	Indigestion treatment – milk of magnesia
Ammonia	Found in the kidney tubules, where it regulates hydrogen ion concentration. 'Cloudy ammonia' is used as a cleaning agent. Also used for perming and colouring hair
Sodium bicarbonate or sodium hydrogencarbonate (baking soda)	Regulates hydrogen ion concentration in blood. Found in toothpaste and indigestion tablets, also used for cooking

Neutralisation

When an acid reacts with a base, it forms salt and water. This reaction is called neutralisation.

$$HCl_{(aq)} + NaOH_{(aq)} \rightarrow NaCl_{(aq)} + H_2O_{(l)}$$
acid   base   salt   water

The stings of many plants and animals contain either acids or bases so we can predict that they can be treated by neutralisation. For example, nettle and ant stings contain an acid called methanoic (formic) acid and this can be neutralised by a base like ammonia which is found in many insect bite ointments, e.g. Afterbite®.

Indigestion is the result of excess hydrochloric acid in the stomach. Excess acid may result over a period of time in peptic ulcers. Heartburn is due to stomach acid refluxing into the oesophagus. The common causes of heartburn are pregnancy, obesity and hiatus hernia. One of the treatments for indigestion and heartburn is to neutralise the acid with indigestion tablets (antacids). Indigestion tablets contain bases such as magnesium hydroxide (milk of magnesia) and aluminium hydroxide. These neutralise the excess stomach acid to produce salt plus water.

$$2HCl_{(aq)} + Mg(OH)_{2(s)} \rightarrow MgCl_{2(aq)} + 2H_2O_{(aq)}$$
stomach   milk of   salt   water
acid   magnesia

When the indigestion tablet contains calcium carbonate or sodium bicarbonate the neutralisation reaction produces salt, water and carbon dioxide gas. The carbon dioxide produced is felt as a 'burp'.

$$2HCl_{(aq)} + CaCO_{3(s)} \rightarrow CaCl_{2(aq)} + H_2O_{(l)} + CO_2\uparrow_{(g)}$$
stomach   calcium   calcium   water   carbon
acid   carbonate   chloride   dioxide

However long-term or excessive usage of indigestion tablets may result in metabolic alkalosis or 'acid rebound' since carbon dioxide released increases the acidity of the stomach.

Salts

Salt is a general name for a compound formed during neutralisation. Table salt (sodium chloride, NaCl) is just one of many compounds that could be classified as a salt. Salts that dissolve in water are electrolytes in solution since they dissociate into their ions. Electrolytes are essential for proper body functioning. Nerve impulses, muscle contraction and the regulation of body fluids depend on the presence of electrolytes. Table 3.3 lists some salts that are used for medical purposes.

The most common salt in the body is calcium phosphate which is found in the bones and teeth. Fizzy drinks and fruit juices are acidic and usually also contain a lot of sugar which can be converted to lactic acid by bacteria in the mouth. Drinking fizzy or fruit drinks may cause

Table 3.3 Medical uses of salts

SALT	MEDICAL APPLICATION
Barium sulphate (barium meal or enema)	X-ray of gastrointestinal tract
Magnesium sulphate (Epsom salts)	Laxative
Calcium chloride	Cardiac injection associated with defibrillation; restoration of electrolyte balance
Sodium chloride	Normal (physiological) saline is used as an intravenous infusion

dental caries (tooth decay) since the acid in them dissolves the calcium salts in the teeth. Frequent brushing and flossing of teeth help to prevent this process.

Strong and weak acids and bases

Strong acid

Hydrochloric acid is a strong acid since it fully dissociates (breaks up) in solution (Fig. 3.1).

$$HCl_{(aq)} \rightarrow H^+_{(aq)} + Cl^-_{(aq)}$$
hydrochloric acid   hydrogen ion   chloride ion

A single-headed arrow ($\rightarrow$) indicates that all the HCl has dissociated into H^+ and Cl^- ions.

Hydrochloric acid, sulphuric acid and nitric acid are all examples of strong acids. These three acids are called the mineral acids.

Weak acid

Ethanoic acid is an organic acid and its common name is vinegar. To be more specific, it is a carboxylic acid (refer to chapter 4). Ethanoic acid is a weak acid since it only partially dissociates in solution (Fig. 3.2). Other examples of weak acids are carbonic acid, citric acid and lactic acid.

$$CH_3COOH_{(aq)} \rightleftharpoons CH_3COO^-_{(aq)} + H^+_{(aq)}$$
ethanoic acid   ethanoate ion   hydrogen ion

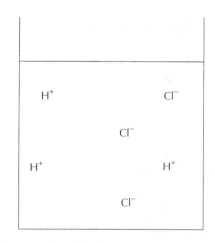

Fig. 3.1 Hydrochloric acid in solution.

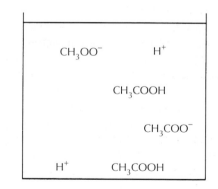

Fig. 3.2 Ethanoic acid in solution.

The two half arrows ($\rightleftharpoons$) indicate that only a few molecules of ethanoic acid have dissociated. Such a reaction is called an equilibrium reaction, and has both the reactant (ethanoic acid)

removal of hydrogen ions
More ethanoic acid will dissociate to give more ethanoate ions and hydrogen ions.
Equilibrium moves to the right to oppose the change.

$$CH_3COOH_{(aq)} \rightleftharpoons CH_3COO^-_{(aq)} \quad + \quad H^+_{(aq)}$$

ethanoic acid   ethanoate ion   hydrogen ion

Equilibrium moves to the left to oppose the change.
The equilibrium is restored by more hydrogen ion combining with ethanoate ion
to reform the acid.
addition of hydrogen ions

Fig. 3.3 Illustration of Le Chatelier's principle.

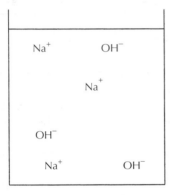

Fig. 3.4 Sodium hydroxide in solution.

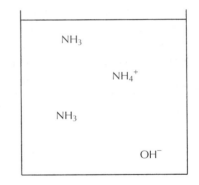

Fig. 3.5 Ammonia in solution.

and products (ethanoate ion and hydrogen ion) present. A dynamic situation exists, since at the same time as the acid is dissociating into its ions, the ions it produces are reuniting to reform the acid.

If anything is done to alter this balance then the equilibrium will move so as to oppose this change. This is known as Le Chatelier's principle (Fig. 3.3).

Strong base

Sodium hydroxide fully dissociates in solution and is a strong base (Fig. 3.4).

$$NaOH_{(aq)} \rightarrow Na^+_{(aq)} + OH^-_{(aq)}$$
sodium hydroxide   sodium ion   hydroxide ion

Other strong bases include potassium hydroxide (KOH), magnesium hydroxide (Mg(OH)$_2$) and calcium hydroxide (Ca(OH)$_2$).

Weak base

Ammonia only partially dissociates in solution and is a weak base (Fig 3.5).

$$NH_{3(g)} + H_2O_{(l)} \rightleftharpoons NH_4^+_{(aq)} + OH^-_{(aq)}$$
ammonia   water   ammonium   hydroxide
                         ion   ion

Some compounds can act as acids and bases these are termed amphoteric; a good example is the bicarbonate ion.

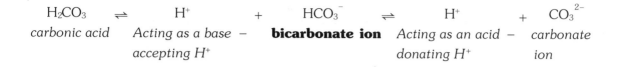

$$H_2CO_3 \rightleftharpoons H^+ + HCO_3^- \rightleftharpoons H^+ + CO_3^{2-}$$

carbonic acid   *Acting as a base –*   **bicarbonate ion**   *Acting as an acid –*   *carbonate*
                  accepting H⁺   *donating H⁺*   *ion*

The bicarbonate ion is also called the hydrogencarbonate ion. The former is the older name and is the name in common usage.

Concentrated and dilute versus strong and weak

Concentrated acids or bases contain a large amount of acid or base in a small amount of water. Dilute acids and bases have a small amount of acid or base in a lot of water. Concentration tells us how much solute is dissolved in the solution and the words concentrated and dilute are used. Strength tells us how much of the acid is dissociated and we use words like strong and weak to indicate acid strengths.

Health and Safety

Acids and bases are corrosive and should never be taken internally. Protective clothing and safety glasses should be worn when handling them in the laboratory. If an acid or base comes in contact with tissue then the area should be washed with plenty of water to dilute the solution. **NEVER** try to neutralise the acid with a base or vice versa.

The pH scale

The pH scale is based on the concentration of hydrogen ions in solution (Fig. 3.6). The more hydrogen ions in solution the lower the pH. Similarly the greater the concentration of hydroxide ions the higher the pH. As a nurse you will measure the pH of body fluids such as blood and urine on a regular basis to detect diseases such as diabetes mellitus.

The pH scale goes from 0 to 14 and it is expressed mathematically as follows:

$$pH = -\log_{10}[H^+]$$

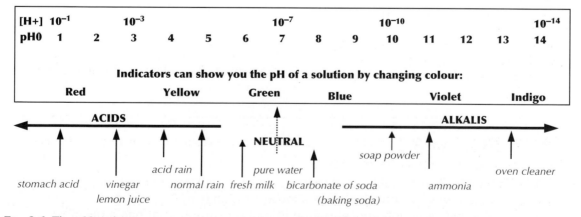

Fig. 3.6 The pH scale

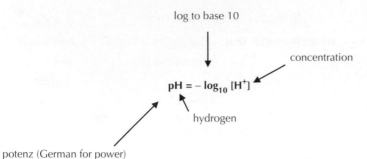

Fig. 3.7 Explanation of pH equation.

Table 3.4 Conversion of hydrogen ion concentration to pH

H$^+$ion concentration (mol/L)	pH	acidic or basic	example
10^{-2}	2	very acidic	sulphuric acid
10^{-5}	5	slightly acidic	black coffee
10^{-7}	7	neutral	pure water
10^{-8}	8	slightly basic	egg white
10^{-14}	14	very basic	sodium hydroxide

The square brackets indicate concentration of hydrogen ions in moles per litre (Fig. 3.7). The normal hydrogen ion concentration of body fluids is very small 40 nmol/L (0.000 000 040 mol/L) so a logarithmic scale is used in order to avoid using a large number of zeros (Table 3.4). The disadvantages of using such a scale are:

(1) one pH unit represents ×10 change in hydrogen ion concentration
(2) increasing hydrogen ion concentration leads to a decreasing pH

At pH 7 the concentration of H$^+$ ions equals the concentration of OH$^-$ ions and the solution is neutral. Pure water has a pH of 7 at 25 °C since water dissociates very slightly to give equal numbers of H$^+$ ions and OH$^-$ ions.

$$H_2O_{(l)} \rightleftharpoons H^+_{(aq)} + OH^-_{(aq)}$$

Solutions with a pH below 7 at 25 °C are acidic. The lower the pH the more acidic the solution.

Solutions with a pH greater than 7 at 25 °C are basic or alkaline. The higher the pH the more basic the solution. Therefore any sub-

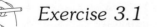 *Exercise 3.1*

a) What is the pH of a 0.1 mol/L hydrochloric acid solution? Would a solution of ethanoic acid of the same concentration have a lower or higher pH?
b) What is the hydrogen ion concentration in a urine sample that has a pH of 5?

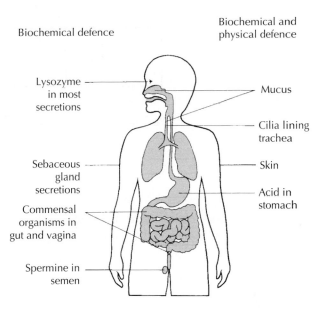

Biochemical defence

Biochemical and physical defence

Lysozyme in most secretions

Mucus

Cilia lining trachea

Sebaceous gland secretions

Skin

Acid in stomach

Commensal organisms in gut and vagina

Spermine in semen

Fig. 3.8 pH values of different body fluids. Source: *Essentials of Physiology*. Lamb, Ingram & Johnston 3rd ed, p. 50.

stance that produces H$^+$ ions or OH$^-$ ions will upset the acid–base balance in the body.

pH of body fluids

Body fluids need to be kept at a constant pH (Fig 3.8). This is because a change in pH will affect all the chemical reactions that occur in the body. Enzymes and other functional proteins, e.g. cytochromes and haemoglobin, have an optimum pH at which they operate best and so are greatly affected by even small changes in pH.

Note, for example that pH values in the stomach and intestine are very different. The enzyme pepsin which breaks down protein in the stomach operates within a pH range of 1.5 to 2.0. If this pH range is not maintained, insufficient protein digestion occurs. The acidic pH in the stomach also neutralises any amylase from saliva that enters the stomach. The pH of the vagina is acidic at 4.5. This not only keeps the vagina healthy by inhibiting the growth of bacteria, but it is also a hostile environment to sperm which are slightly alkaline. The pH of the vagina changes with age, being acidic during

the reproductive years. Before puberty and after the menopause it is slightly alkaline.

The normal pH range for blood is 7.35–7.45 (see Fig. 3.9). The range of blood pH compatible with life is only 7.0–7.8. The term alkalosis is used when the pH of arterial blood rises above 7.45. The patient would be described as alkalotic. Conversely a pH of below 7.35 is known as acidosis. (This term is used because the blood is more acidic than it should be. It does not matter in this special case that the actual pH is above neutral). The patient would be described as acidotic. Small changes in blood pH can be fatal, a patient who has a blood pH of 7.25 or 7.7 is likely to be in a coma.

Hydrogen ions are being continually produced by the body. The two main sources are:

- Cellular metabolism, e.g. anaerobic respiration produces lactic acid; fat metabolism produces ketone bodies. Also phosphorus and sulphur present in amino acids and lipids are metabolised to phosphoric and sulphuric acids. These acids are often referred to as the 'non-volatile' or 'fixed' acids.
- Cellular respiration – in 24 hours some 10 000–20 000 mmol of carbon dioxide is

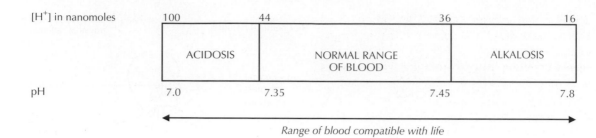

| [H⁺] in nanomoles | 100 | 44 | | 36 | 16 |

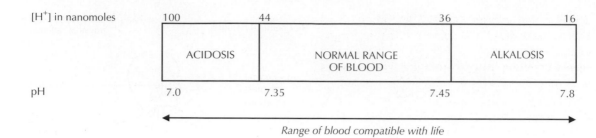

Fig. 3.9 pH of blood.

produced and changed to carbonic acid before it is excreted by the lungs.

This means that there must be systems within the body which regulate acid–base levels.

These body systems are:

- chemical buffer systems
- respiratory regulatory systems (the lungs)
- renal regulatory systems (kidneys).

All these systems work together as a team to regulate body pH. Initially we will look at them working individually, and then together.

Chemical buffers

Buffers are chemical solutions which resist changes in pH on addition of either an acid or base. Buffer solutions consist of:
either a solution of a weak acid and its salt, for example carbonic acid and sodium bicarbonate **or** a solution of a weak base and its salt, for example ammonia solution and ammonium chloride.

If pH is decreasing, then the salt (sodium bicarbonate) acts as a base accepting any hydrogen ions added to the solution. If pH is increasing, the weak acid (carbonic acid) will donate hydrogen ions to the solution; so pH changes are 'buffered'. For the weak base/salt buffer system the situation is reversed.

In general buffers react by releasing or taking up hydrogen ions:

$\Leftarrow$ decrease in hydrogen ion concentration

$$H^+ + Buffer^- \rightleftharpoons HBuffer$$

increase in hydrogen ion concentration $\Rightarrow$

Note the hydrogen ions are not removed from the body they are just 'trapped' by the buffer. The main chemical buffer systems found in the body are:

- bicarbonate buffer system
- phosphate buffer system
- protein buffer system

All the buffer systems work together to restore pH in a fraction of a second, but there is a limit to the extent to which pH can be kept constant by a buffer. This will depend on the reservoir of buffer present and is known as the 'buffering capacity'. If large amounts of acid or base are added then the buffer system will not be able to cope.

Bicarbonate buffer system

The bicarbonate buffer system is the major extracellular buffer and is responsible for maintaining blood pH. Carbon dioxide formed during cell respiration dissolves in water (plasma) to form carbonic acid. This carbonic acid then partially dissociates to give hydrogen ions and bicarbonate ions. The bicarbonate ion acts as the hydrogen ion acceptor. When hydrogen ions are added to the body, for example lactic acid which is formed during exercise, the bicarbonate ion combines with the hydrogen ions from the lactic acid forming carbonic acid. The carbonic acid acts as the hydrogen ion donor. When hydrogen ions are lost from the body, as in the case of severe vomiting, more carbonic acid dissociates to give hydrogen ions and bicarbonate ions. The normal ratio of bicarbonate to carbonic acid is 20 : 1 (see euqation 1).

The bicarbonate system buffers 90% of the hydrogen ions in blood and is important since the amount of carbon dioxide and bicarbonate ion can also be regulated by the lungs and the kidneys respectively. The amount of bicarbonate ion available for buffering is known as the alkaline reserve.

Phosphate buffer system

This is similar to the bicarbonate buffer system. The sodium salts of dihydrogen phosphate and monohydrogen phosphate act as the weak acid and base respectively (see equation 2).

The phosphate buffer mainly buffers the intracellular fluid and the kidney tubules, it

therefore does not buffer blood but is an important buffer for urine.

Protein buffer system

Proteins are long chains of amino acids joined together. Amino acids contain a basic amino group (NH_2) and an acidic group (COOH). Three forms of amino acids exist depending on pH (see equation 3).

Protein buffers are very complex systems and they buffer the intracellular fluid and plasma. The protein haemoglobin performs two specialised functions, it transports oxygen to the tissue and it also buffers hydrogen ions in transit from the cells to the lungs.

Haemoglobin buffer system

Carbon dioxide diffuses into the erythrocyte (red blood cell). Inside the cell, carbon dioxide is converted to carbonic acid in the presence of

---

Equation box

Bicarbonate buffer system

$$\Leftarrow \text{addition of hydrogen ions} \quad CO_2 + H_2O \rightleftharpoons H_2CO_3 \rightleftharpoons H^+ + HCO_3^- \quad \text{loss of hydrogen ions} \Rightarrow$$

carbon dioxide   carbon water   acid   hydrogen ion   bicarbonate ion   (1)

Phosphare buffer system

Addition of hydrogen ions $\Rightarrow$ H^+ + HPO_4^{2-} $\rightleftharpoons$ $H_2PO_4^-$ $\Leftarrow$ loss of hydrogen ions

hydrogen ion   monohydrogen phosphate ion   dihydrogen phosphate ion   (2)

weak base   **weak acid**

Protein buffer system

$$H_3N^+-CH_2-COOH \rightleftharpoons H_3N^+-CH_2-COO^- \rightleftharpoons H_2N-CH_2-COO^-$$

acidic   *Zwitter ion–neutral*   *basic*   (3)

Haemoglobin buffer system

Carbonic anhydrase CO_2 + H_2O $\rightleftharpoons$ H_2CO_3 $\rightleftharpoons$ H^+ + HCO_3^-

carbon dioxide   water   carbonic acid   hydrogen ion   bicarbonate ion   (4)

H^+ + HbO_2^- $\rightleftharpoons$ HHb + O_2

hydrogen ion   oxyhaemoglobin   reduced haemoglobin   oxygen   (5)

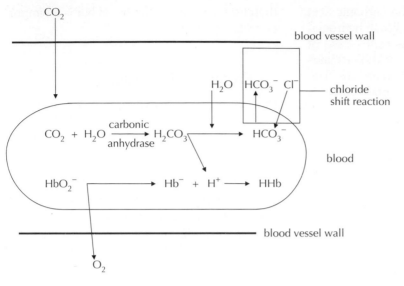

Fig. 3.10 Haemoglobin buffer system.

the enzyme carbonic anhydrase. The carbonic acid partially dissociates to give hydrogen ions and bicarbonate ions (see equation 4).

Haemoglobin then combines with these hydrogen ions to form reduced haemoglobin (see equation 5).

This reaction occurs because reduced haemoglobin is a weaker acid than oxyhaemoglobin and carbonic acid and therefore forms a stronger bond to hydrogen. Therefore when oxygen is released the hydrogen ions produced by the uptake of carbon dioxide are 'trapped' by the haemoglobin, preventing any change in the pH.

Once formed in the erythrocyte the bicarbonate ions diffuse out into the plasma, where they become part of the alkaline reserve and buffer hydrogen ions. At the same time as bicarbonate ions are diffusing out of the erythrocyte, chloride ions are diffusing in. This occurs to maintain cell neutrality or charge balance and is known as the chloride shift reaction (Fig. 3.10).

In the alveoli of the lungs the whole process is reversed and carbon dioxide and water are removed by breathing.

Ammonia buffer system

Ammonia is formed in the tubule cells of the kidneys from the breakdown of amino acids. The ammonia diffuses into the tubules, where it buffers hydrogen ions in the renal filtrate, forming ammonium ions. The ammonium ions are then excreted in the urine which prevents the urine becoming too acidic.

$$NH_3 \quad + \quad H^+ \quad \rightarrow \quad NH_4^+$$
ammonia   hydrogen ion   ammonium ion

Respiratory regulation of pH

Changes in breathing (ventilation) can dramatically change pH. If ventilation is doubled or halved it can change the pH by 0.2 pH units. In a healthy person carbon dioxide is produced at the rate of 10 mmol per min, this is expelled from the lungs as fast as it is formed in the tissue. The rate of ventilation is precisely regulated to the level of Pco_2 and hydrogen ion (pH) concentration in arterial blood (Pco_2 indicates the partial pressure of carbon dioxide, in arterial blood). These levels are monitored by peripheral (carotid + aortic bodies) chemoreceptors and the central chemoreceptors in the medulla which are sensitive to changes in the pH of cerebrospinal fluid (chemoreceptors respond to chemical changes in their surroundings). They respond by changing the rate and depth of ventilation. The normal value for P_{CO_2} is 4.7–6.0 kPa or 35–45 mmHg. Respiratory acidosis occurs when there is accumulation of carbon dioxide in the blood and P_{CO_2} increases above normal, i.e. >6 kPa. Respiratory alkalosis occurs when carbon dioxide is lost from the blood and P_{CO_2} decreases below normal, i.e. <4.7 kPa.

Regulation of pH by ventilation occurs by two mechanisms:

a) Increasing P_{CO_2} or H^+ ion concentration means that pH will decrease. As a result the respiratory centre in the medulla is stimulated and breathing becomes deeper and faster (hyperventilation). This removes the carbon dioxide and shifts the equilibrium in the equation below to the left and restores values to normal. This is also a negative feedback mechanism (Fig. 3.11).

$$H_2O + CO_2 \rightleftharpoons H_2CO_3 \rightleftharpoons H^+ + HCO_3^-$$

b) Decreasing P_{CO_2} or H^+ ion concentration means that pH will increase. As a result the respiratory centre in the medulla is depressed and breathing becomes shallower and slower (hypoventilation). The equilibrium in the equation above is pushed to the right causing carbon dioxide to accumulate thus restoring normal values. This is also a negative feedback mechanism (Fig. 3.11).

The respiratory system reacts slower than the buffer systems, 1–3 minutes compared with seconds. However the respiratory system, unlike the buffer systems, actually removes hydrogen ions from the body and so there is no limit to the capacity of the respiratory system.

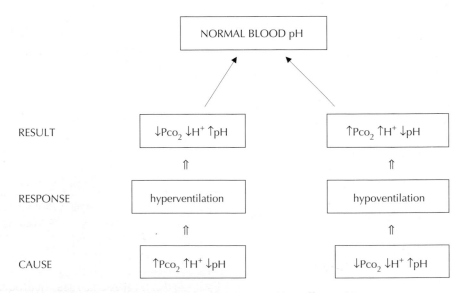

Fig. 3.11 Negative feedback mechanism, showing how respiration affects pH.

■ ■ *Renal regulation of pH*

℅ *Activity*

Look at the diagram of the nephron (Fig. 3.12). What are the main parts of the nephron? How does the blood flow through the kidneys? Where does filtration occur in the nephron? What is the tubular system? If you are unable to answer these questions you must find a physiology text book and read the chapter on the urinary (renal) system.

There are about 1.3 million nephrons in each kidney. The functions of the nephron are filtration, secretion and reabsorption (Fig. 3.13). The kidneys regulate pH by selectively removing or returning ions and other products to the blood. It filters 1.2 L of blood per minute.

Buffers work within seconds and the respiratory system within minutes but the renal system takes hours or even days. Compare how many times you go to the toilet a day with how many times you breathe a day. Like the respiratory system the kidneys remove acids and bases from the body and again there is no limit to the capacity of the system.

The kidneys are responsible for getting rid of the fixed acids such as lactic acid and phosphoric acid formed during metabolism. A drop in pH due to accumulation of these acids is called metabolic acidosis. Regulation of the bicarbonate ion is only done by the kidneys. The reabsorption of bicarbonate ions enables renewal of that buffer system. Accumulation of bicarbonate ions in the blood results in metabolic alkalosis. During metabolic

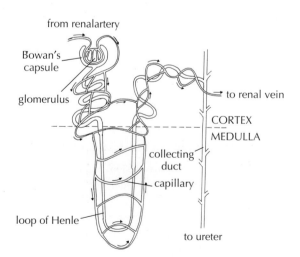

Fig. 3.12 A nephron – the functional unit of the kidney.

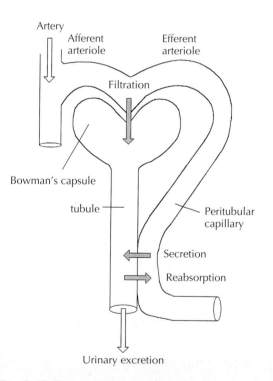

Fig. 3.13 Function of the nephron.

acidosis, the kidneys maintain pH by secreting hydrogen ions and reabsorbing bicarbonate ions. During metabolic alkalosis the opposite happens.

When the balancing act no longer works

Normal acid–base values for arterial blood

pH	7.35–7.45
P_{CO_2}	4.7–6.0 kPa or 35–45 mm Hg
$[HCO_3^-]$	21–30 mmol/L
Base excess	−2 → +2

In respiratory acidosis carbon dioxide accumulates in the blood due to hypoventilation and this is reflected in the falling blood pH and rising P_{CO_2} values. Respiratory alkalosis is rarely caused by disease (pathological). Carbon dioxide is removed from the blood due to hyperventilation, causing blood pH to rise and P_{CO_2} to fall. Metabolic abnormalities are caused by all acid–base imbalances, except those caused by carbon dioxide. Metabolic acidosis is recognised by falling blood pH and $[HCO_3^-]$ levels, whilst metabolic alkalosis is recognised by increasing pH and $[HCO_3^-]$ levels Figs 3.14 and 3.15.

The normal value of the base excess is zero. In metabolic alkalosis it is positive and in metabolic acidosis it is negative – it will not be used further in this book.

Activity

Use the flow charts to answer the following questions:
a) A patient has been vomiting severely over a period of time. What acid has been lost from the body? How does this affect the blood pH? What treatment could be given to such a patient? What type of acid–base imbalance is the patient likely to be suffering from?
b) A patient has taken several packets of indigestion tablets over a short period of time. What do indigestion tablets contain? How does this affect the blood pH? What treatment could be given to such a patient? What type of acid–base imbalance is the patient likely to be suffering from?

Let us look at some acid–base values from blood laboratory results:

Patient 1
pH 7.25
P_{CO_2} 5.6 kPa

Patient 2
pH 7.52
P_{CO_2} 3.2 kPa

$[HCO_3^-]$ 19 mmol/L
pH is low – acidosis
P_{CO_2} is normal
$[HCO_3^-]$ is low
Conclusion metabolic acidosis

$[HCO_3^-]$ 23 mmol/L
pH is high – alkalosis
P_{CO_2} is low
$[HCO_3^-]$ is normal
Conclusion respiratory alkalosis

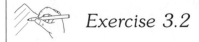 ## Exercise 3.2

Patient 3 has the following acid–base values. What acid–base imbalance is indicated by the blood laboratory results?   pH 7.30 P_{CO_2} 7.8 kPa $[HCO_3^-]$ 24 mmol/L

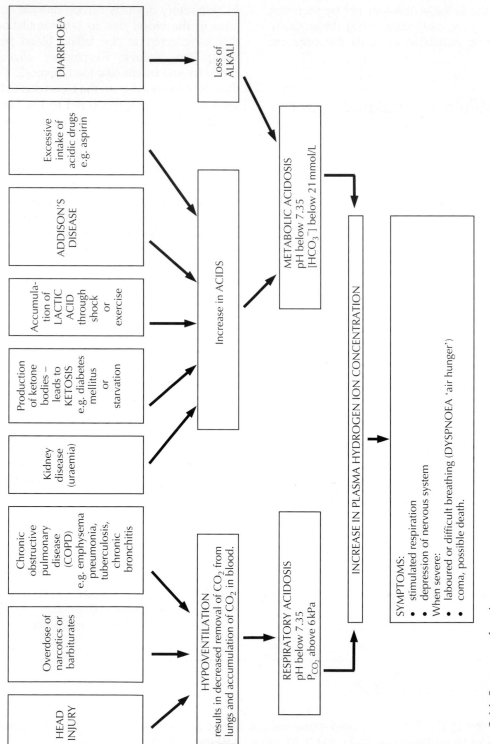

Fig. 3.14 Summary of acidosis.

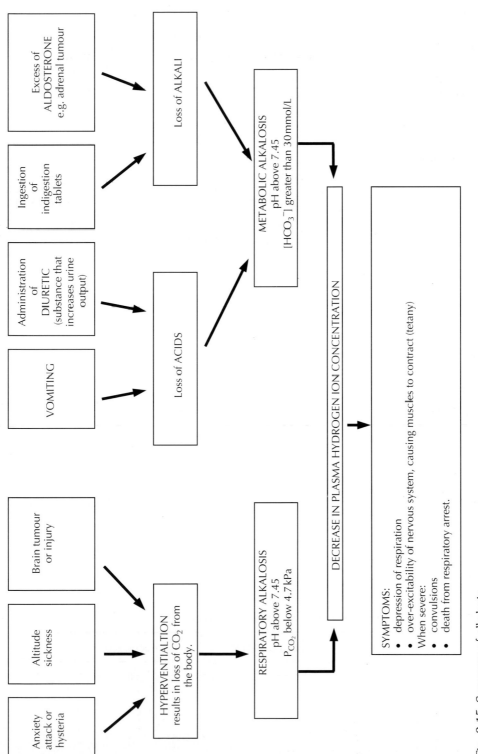

Fig. 3.15 Summary of alkalosis.

Compensation – systems working together

The buffer system, the respiratory system and the renal system work together to maintain the acid–base balance in the body. It must be remembered that in a homeostatic system if one system is disturbed or not working properly, then the other systems will try to compensate for it. The respiratory and renal compensations can be seen in changes in Pco_2 and bicarbonate values of the blood. Respiratory compensation involves changes in ventilation rate and depth whilst renal compensation involves changes in blood levels of the bicarbonate ion. A summary of acid–base disturbances is given in Table 3.5.

Let us look at some examples of compensation:

Patient 4
pH 7.48
Pco_2 6.8 kPa
$[HCO_3^-]$ 33 mmol/L
pH – high, alkalosis
Pco_2 high (this is the cause of respiratory acidosis not alkalosis)
$[HCO_3^-]$ high

metabolic alkalosis compensated for by respiratory acidosis

Patient 5
pH 7.33
Pco_2 7.5 kPa
$[HCO_3^-]$ 35 mmol/L
pH – low, acidosis
Pco_2 high (this is a case of respiratory acidosis)
$[HCO_3^-]$ high (retention of HCO_3^- by kidneys to restore pH)

respiratory acidosis compensated for by metabolic alkalosis

Exercise 3.3

Patient 6 has the following acid–base values. What acid–base imbalance is indicated by the blood laboratory results?   pH 7.32 Pco_2 4.3 kPa $[HCO_3^-]$ 18 mmol/L

Summary

- Acids are hydrogen ion donors whilst bases are hydrogen ion acceptors
- Strong acids and bases are fully dissociated in solution. Weak acids and bases are only partially dissociated in solution
- pH scale is a scale of hydrogen ion concentration and goes from 0 to 14
- Acids have a pH below 7, bases have a pH above 7. A pH of 7 is neutral at 25 °C
- Buffers resist changes in pH
- The pH of the body is maintained by the kidneys, lungs and the buffer systems of the body
- Acidosis results if the blood becomes too acidic, alkalosis results if the blood becomes too basic

Table 3.5 Summary of acid–base disturbances

	Uncompensated			Compensated		
	pH	$[HCO_3^-]$	Pco_2	pH	$[HCO_3^-]$	Pco_2
Metabolic acidosis	↓	↓	–	↓	↓	↓
Metabolic alkalosis	↑	↑	–	↑	↑	↑
Respiratory acidosis	↓	–	↑	↓	↑	↑
Respiratory alkalosis	↑	–	↓	↑	↓	↓

- One system will compensate for another system to maintain homeostasis.

Review Questions

3.1.   Place the following household substances in order of increasing pH: baking soda, fruit juice, oven cleaner, fresh milk, soap powder and black coffee.

3.2.   A pregnant woman has heartburn. On her doctor's advice she is taking indigestion tablets containing sodium bicarbonate. What are the products formed when the excess acid is neutralised by the tablets?

3.3.   A patient has suffered an asthma attack. The patient's blood laboratory results are given below. Determine the cause of the acid–base imbalance.

pH 7.5

P_{CO_2} 3.5 kPa

$[HCO_3^-]$ 22 mmol/L

3.4.   Explain why a paper bag held over the mouth and nose of a person hyperventilating would help to alleviate the symptoms.

3.5.   A patient's blood test results are given below. Identify the cause of the acid–base imbalance.

pH 7.30

P_{CO_2} 4.3 kPa

$[HCO_3^-]$ 18 mmol/L

Further reading

Bray, J.J., Cragg, P.A., MacKnight, A.D.C. & Mills, R.G. (1999). *Lecture Notes on Human Physiology* (4th edn). Blackwell Science Ltd, Oxford.

Marieb, E.N. (2000). *Human Anatomy and Physiology* (5th edn). Benjamin Cummings, Redwood City, California.

Tortora, G.J. & Grabowska, S.R. (1999). *Principles of Anatomy and Physiology* (9th edn). John Wiley & Sons Ltd, Chichester.

Chapter Four
BIOMOLECULES

Learning objectives

By the end of this chapter the reader will be able to:
- Describe the structure of carbohydrates, fats and proteins
- List the functional groups of carbohydrates, fats and proteins
- Describe the digestion and absorption of carbohydrates, fats and proteins
- Describe the structure of a nucleotide
- List the differences between RNA and DNA.

Introduction

Biomolecules are any molecules large or small found in living organisms and manufactured by the cell. The biomolecules – carbohydrates (starch and sugars), lipids (fats and oils), proteins and nucleic acids (the hereditary material) all contain carbon. Biomolecules also contain specific groups of atoms (functional groups) which are responsible for their structure, reactivity and function.

Organic chemistry

Organic chemistry is the study of carbon compounds. All living things contain carbon – you contain about 18% carbon. Originally the word 'organic' meant 'obtained from living things' but today thousands of organic compounds such as drugs and plastics are made artificially in laboratories.

There are millions of organic compounds and they are therefore placed in families or homologous series. The fact there are so many of them is due to the unique properties of the carbon atom:

1. It will form four covalent bonds with other atoms:

$$-\overset{|}{\underset{|}{C}}-$$

2. Carbon atoms join together readily to form both chains, e.g. fats, and rings, e.g. steroids and carbohydrates.

$$CH_3 — CH_2 — CH_2 — CH_2 — CH_2 — CH_3$$

chain

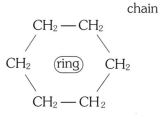

3. Even if organic compounds have the same molecular formula (number of atoms), they may have a different structural formula (different shape) – these are called isomers.

Structural formula	**Molecular formula**
$CH_3 — CH_2 — CH_2 — CH_3$	C_4H_{10}
$CH_3 — \underset{\underset{CH_3}{\vert}}{CH} — CH_3$	C_4H_{10}

Sometimes the different shape that isomers have are important in determining whether they are active within the body or not.

Carbohydrates

Carbohydrates contain only carbon, hydrogen and oxygen. They are called carbohydrates because the ratio of hydrogen to oxygen in them is $2:1$, which is the same as the ratio in water. The word saccharide indicates a sugar with the name of the sugar ending in -ose. All carbohydrates contain the $-OH$ hydroxyl functional group and belong to the alcohol family. Historically they were called the sugar alcohols.

Carbohydrates are divided into three groups depending on their size and solubility:

* Monosaccharides – 'one sugar units' and are soluble in water. They are the building block of all other carbohydrates (Fig. 4.1)

Monosaccharide: one unit

Disaccharide: two units

Polysaccharide: many units

STARCH

Amylose

Amylopectin

CELLULOSE

Hydrogen bonds

20% unbranched twisted into helix

80% branched helix; less highly branched than glycogen

Hydrogen bonds link chains together giving cellulose its strength and making it suitable as a structural material

GLYCOGEN

Highly branched; the many branch endings can be hydrolysed to give the body almost immediate access to glucose

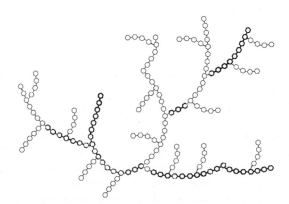

Fig. 4.1 Structural relationship between various carbohydrates.

- Disaccharides – 'two sugar units' and are soluble in water (Fig. 4.1)
- Polysachharide – 'many sugar units' and are insoluble in water (Fig. 4.1).

Monosaccharides (simple sugars)

Monosaccharides exist in both an 'open-chain' form and as rings. These two forms readily interconvert and in solution the 'open chain form' closes to form the more stable ring structure.

Only three monosaccharides commonly occur in the diet. These are glucose (blood sugar or dextrose), fructose (fruit sugar) and galactose. Each can be represented by the molecular formula $C_6H_{12}O_6$ and are called hexoses since they contain six carbon atoms. Monosaccharides with five carbon atoms are called pentoses, e.g. ribose and deoxyribose (Fig. 4.2).

Fructose, galactose and glucose are isomers – that is they have the same molecular formula but a different structural formula (Fig. 4.2). This means they will have different chemical properties. On close inspection of the structures of glucose and fructose you will see that they contain different functional groups. Glucose contains the aldehyde functional group (Fig. 4.3) and is called an aldose.

Fructose has a ketone as a functional group (Fig. 4.4) and is a ketose:

All monosaccharides are reducing sugars since they readily react with reagents such as Benedict's and Fehling's solutions. They reduce these blue solutions to a brick red solid, this test is used by biologists in the laboratory to identify reducing sugars.

Historically, Benedict's and Fehling's solutions were used in hospitals to test for glucose in blood and urine. Glucose is used by the cells as a source of energy. The normal value for blood glucose is 3.5–5.5 mmol/L. In diseases such as diabetes mellitus the concentration of glucose in the blood is higher than normal – hyperglycaemia and the excess glucose is

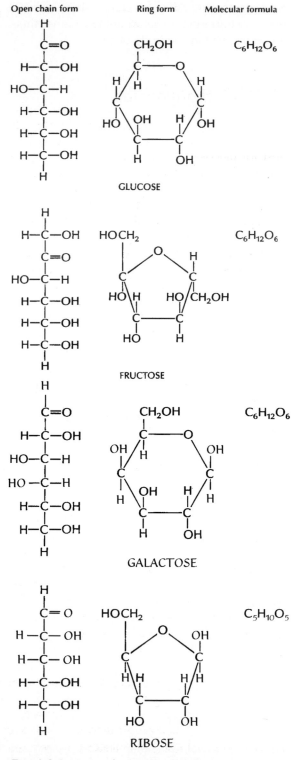

Fig. 4.2 Isomers of monosaccharides.

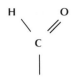

Fig. 4.3. Aldehyde functional group.

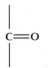

Fig. 4.4 Ketone functional group.

excreted in the urine (glycosuria). Glucose is not normally found in the urine. Today nurses test for glucose in urine with urinalysis reagent strips which change colour depending on the concentration of glucose, e.g. Clinistix® or Labstix®. Blood testing gives a direct measure of blood glucose. A sample of blood is obtained by pricking the finger pulp placing the blood on a reagent strip and then into a glucometer, e.g. Glucotrend® which gives a digital readout. A new strip for each sample should be used and the instructions read before use. Hands should be washed, with soap and water only, to remove any substances such as alcohol, that could interfere with the glucometer reading.

Monosaccharides contain a large number of –OH (hydroxyl) functional groups. The hydroxyl group is able to hydrogen bond with water making monosaccharides soluble in water. The presence of the –OH group on adjacent carbon atoms in the molecule is also thought to give sugars their 'sweet' taste.

Disaccharides

Important disaccharides in the diet include sucrose (cane or table sugar), lactose (milk sugar) and maltose (malt sugar). Lactose and maltose are reducing sugars, but sucrose is known as a non-reducing sugar. Disaccharides are formed when two monosaccharides are joined with the loss of a water molecule in a condensation reaction. The general reaction is below.

The covalent bond holding the two monosaccharide units together is called a glycosidic bond – this –C–O–C– bond is the ether functional group (Fig. 4.5).

Disaccharides are too large to be absorbed directly from the intestine and they must be digested into monosaccharides before absorption. This occurs by hydrolysis (hydro = water, lysis = splitting). Hydrolysis is the reverse of condensation and involves the addition of water usually in the presence of enzymes, which act as catalysts.

Polysaccharides

Polysaccharides are long chains of many repeating sugar molecules. Such structures are called polymers or macromolecules. Polysaccharides can contain up to 26 000 glucose molecules and are fairly insoluble in water due to their size. The three most important polysaccharides are cellulose, starch and glycogen.

Cellulose (fibre)

Cellulose occurs in all plants as part of their cell wall and it is the most abundant organic compound on Earth. It is made up of long straight chains of glucose molecules and is not digested since humans lack the enzyme cellulase. Cellulose (Fig. 4.1) is hygroscopic, that is, it picks up water and makes the stool bulkier and softer to

$$\text{monosaccharide} + \overset{\text{condensation}}{\text{monosaccharide}} \rightleftharpoons \text{disaccharide} + \text{water}$$

e.g.   hydrolysis
glucose + fructose $\rightleftharpoons$ sucrose + water
glucose + glucose $\rightleftharpoons$ maltose + water
glucose + galactose $\rightleftharpoons$ lactose + water

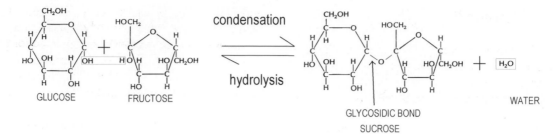

Fig. 4.5 Synthesis of a disaccharide.

expel. Excess fibre can lead to flatulence (farts) caused by bacteria in the large intestine fermenting the undigested cellulose and food to release gases such as methane and hydrogen sulphide (the latter causes the smell). A high-fibre diet can help prevent cancers of the large intestine.

Glycogen

Excess glucose is stored as glycogen (animal starch) in humans and animals. Glycogen is found in the liver and the skeletal muscles and is made up of many glucose molecules linked together in highly branched chains (Fig. 4.1). This branched arrangement permits rapid hydrolysis of glycogen. Roughly one-third of the body's stored glycogen is found in the liver, with two-thirds in the skeletal muscle. Glucose is converted to glycogen in the presence of insulin in the liver cells (hepatocytes), this process is known as glycogenesis. The reverse process (glycogen to glucose) is known as glycogenolysis. There is enough carbohydrate stored as glycogen to provide for about a day's energy

needs and glucose for about an hour's energy needs.

Glycogen is also stored in skeletal muscle, this can be converted to glucose by the action of the enzyme muscle phosphorylase. Glucose produced in the muscle in this way is used only to provide energy for muscle contraction. If the glycogen stores are full then glucose can be converted to fat and stored in the adipose tissue.

Starch

Plants store excess glucose as starch – long, straight (amylose) or branched (amylopectin) chains of hundreds or thousands of glucose molecules linked together (Fig. 4.1). Starches and glycogen are good storage substances since both are only sparingly soluble in water. Starch molecules accumulate to form starch granules and are visible in many plant cells, e.g. potato. Carbohydrates are the preferred dietary source of energy. Starches account for approximately 60% of the total carbohydrate intake in the average British diet and sugars account for 40%.

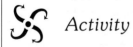 Activity

Iodine is used to treat cuts and you can buy some at the chemist. Test the following foods with a drop of iodine. Note which foods contain starch. The test for starch is iodine, the brown solution of iodine turns blue/black in the presence of starch.

a) bread   b) meat
c) crisps   d) butter

Lipids

A wide range of biomolecules are classified as lipids because they are soluble in other lipids (lipophilic) and organic solvents such as alcohols, but insoluble in water. There are four classes of lipids:

- triglycerides
- phospholipids
- steroids
- prostaglandins.

Triglycerides (neutral fats)

Triglycerides are the fats found in the diet and are the richest source of dietary energy. Triglycerides are made up of two sub-units – glycerol and fatty acids. Glycerol contains the –OH functional group and is an alcohol.

Fatty acids are long chains of carbon and hydrogen atoms that contain the carboxylic acid functional group (Fig. 4.6). Because of these long hydrophobic carbon chains fats are insoluble in water. If the carbons in the chain are linked only by single bonds (C–C) then the fatty acid is said to be saturated. If the carbons in the chain are linked by double bonds (C=C) then the fatty acid is said to be unsaturated. The more double bonds present in the molecule the more likely it is that the fatty acid will be an oil (Figs. 4.7 & 4.8). Stearic acid is saturated and can be considered as a straight cylinder which can pack together tightly to form a solid at room temperature. Oleic acid is monounsaturated (contains only one double bond) and arachidonic acid is polyunsaturated (contains many double bonds). Unsaturated fatty acids are bent cylinders and due to this they cannot pack close together and are liquid at room temperature. Unsaturated fatty acids tend to be of plant origin

and liquid, e.g. olive oil, whilst saturated fats tend to be of animal origin and solid, e.g. butter.

Polyunsaturated fatty acids are needed for the manufacture of cell membranes and substances such as prostaglandins. The body cannot synthesise these fatty acids so they are sometimes

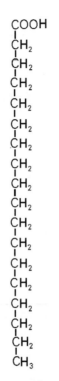

Fig. 4.7 Saturated fatty acid.

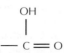

Fig. 4.6 Carboxylic acid functional group.

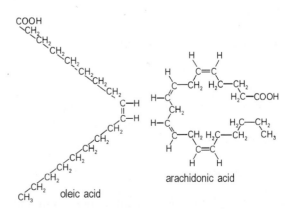

Fig. 4.8 Unsaturated fatty acids.

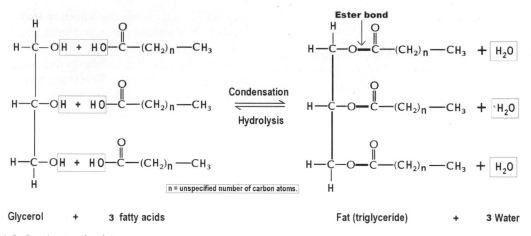

Fig. 4.9 Synthesis of a fat.

referred to as essential fatty acids as we must obtain them in our diet.

Triglycerides are formed when three fatty acids combine with one glycerol molecule with the elimination of water to form an E-shaped triglyceride (Fig. 4.9). Triglycerides contain the ester functional group (Fig. 4.10).

For any triglyceride the fatty acids can all be the same or can be different. Palmitic, oleic and stearic acids make up about 80% of fatty acids found in triglycerides.

Phospholipids

Similar in structure to triglycerides except they contain only two fatty acids, the third fatty acid being replaced by a phosphorus-containing group. Phospholipids contain two distinct areas and are found in cell membranes (Fig. 4.11).

Due to the presence of the polar/non-polar areas phospholipids tend to arrange themselves in a double layer or bilayer. The phospholipid cell membrane has a protective function and is vital in transporting substances into and out of the cell.

Steroids

Steroids are fat-soluble compounds. Different chains of atoms extend out from the rings and

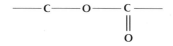

Fig. 4.10 Ester functional group.

the nature of these chains determines the steroid formed (Fig. 4.12). Among the important steroids in the body are the sex hormones, bile salts, corticosteroids and cholesterol.

Cholesterol is an important component of cell membranes and is used by the body to synthesise other steroids, e.g. oestrogen. Cholesterol is insoluble in water and to be transported in blood it must bind to a special protein called an 'apoprotein' to produce a lipoprotein. There are three classes of lipoproteins:

- high density lipoproteins (HDLs) – little cholesterol combined with a large amount of protein, cholesterol is transported to the liver to be excreted in this form
- low density lipoproteins (LDLs) and very low density proteins (VLDLs) – have lots of cholesterol combined with a little protein, cholesterol is transported to the cells and tissues in this form

LDLs and VLDLs are connected to the development of atherosclerosis (narrowing of the blood vessels). Atherosclerosis occurs due to

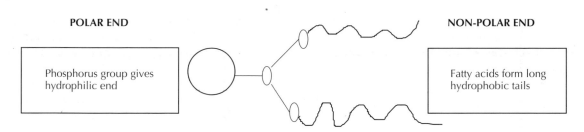

Fig. 4.11 Diagrammatic representation of a phospholipid.

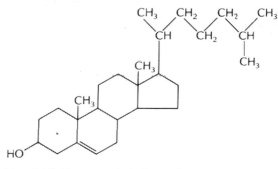

Fig. 4.12 The steroid cholesterol.

excess cholesterol, fibrin, other lipids and calcium being deposited on the walls of blood vessels, particularly the coronary arteries to produce areas or plaques called atheroma. These plaques narrow the blood vessels and reduce blood flow. A range of cardiovascular diseases (diseases of the heart and blood vessels) are associated with this condition.

- ischaemic heart disease – myocardial infarction (heart attack)
- cerebrovascular disease – cerebrovascular accident (CVA or stroke)
- peripheral vascular disease – due to lack of oxygen, e.g. painful limbs.

A high ratio of LDL to HDL (too much LDL) is associated with an increased risk of cardiovascular disease. Raised cholesterol levels are associated with:

- Inherited genetic defects in LDL production
- Lifestyle – smoking, over-weight, stress and diet (eating animal fats).

It is known that the ratio of HDL to LDL is increased in the blood of people who are vegetarians or non-smokers and those who exercise.

$\mathcal{S}$ *Activity*

Look at your own diet, do you have a diet that is high in saturated fats? Do you grill or fry your food? Do you use unsaturated fats in the diet? Is there a family history of heart disease? Do you smoke?

Prostaglandins

Prostaglandins are derived from fatty acids and are found in all body tissues where they act as chemical mediators (Fig. 4.13). They are synthesised in response to a stimulus and act quickly and locally and are then broken down. Prostaglandins may raise or lower blood pres-

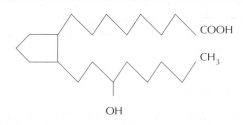

Fig. 4.13 General structure of prostaglandins.

sure, regulate blood clotting and play a role in temperature regulation and pain perception. Prostaglandins are also used as drugs, e.g. vaginal pessaries containing prostaglandins are used to ripen the cervix as well as induce labour. Aspirin prevents the formation of prostaglandins and therefore can be used as analgesics and antipyretics.

Proteins

Proteins like polysaccharides are polymers or macromolecules. The building blocks of proteins are amino acids.

Amino acids

Amino acids have two functional groups the amino $-NH_2$ and the carboxylic acid group $-COOH$ (Fig. 4.14).

When a protein is eaten it is digested to give amino acids, which are absorbed and used by the body to make other proteins in the body. Twenty different amino acids are commonly found in dietary proteins. Of these about 10 are non-essential since they can be made by the body. The remainder are essential amino acids since they have to be provided in the diet (Table 4.1). In children, unlike adults, histidine is also an essential amino acid since they cannot synthesise enough to meet their needs.

The amount of protein in food varies considerably. If the food contains all the essential amino acids it is classed as a complete protein, if it is low in the essential amino acids it is classed as an incomplete protein. The amino acid that is in shortest supply in relation to need is called the limiting amino acid. In general, proteins from animals, e.g. meat, eggs and fish are complete proteins. Proteins from plant sources tend to lack certain amino acids, e.g. lysine is the limiting amino acid in wheat. However, if a varied diet is eaten, even if a person is a vegan or vegetarian, all the essential amino acids will be provided.

R is different for every amino acid, in the simplest amino acid glycine R is a hydrogen atom

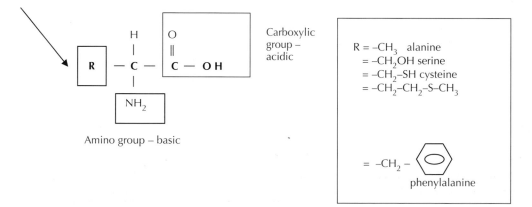

Fig. 4.14 General formula of amino acids.

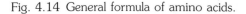 ## Exercise 4.1

Draw the structures of the amino acids glycine, alanine and phenylalanine.

Table 4.1 Essential amino acids

| Leucine | Threonine | Methionine | Arginine | Tryptophan |
| Lysine | Valine | Phenylalanine | (Histidine) | Isoleucine |

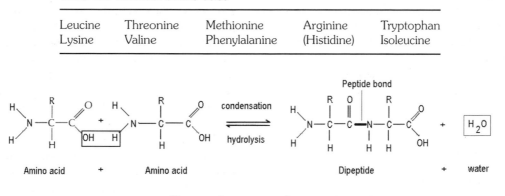

R = various organic groups

Fig. 4.15 Synthesis of a dipeptide.

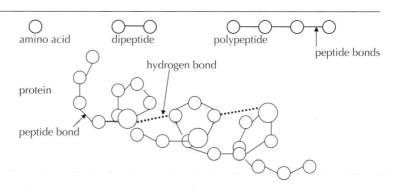

Fig. 4.16 Structural relationship between amino acids, peptides and proteins.

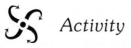 *Proteins, polypeptides and dipeptides*

When two amino acids are linked together by a peptide bond a dipeptide is formed (Fig. 4.15).

Polypeptides contain 10 or more amino acids linked together by peptide bonds. Proteins contain 50 or more amino acids joined together by peptide bonds, however most proteins contain thousands of amino acids as they are macromolecules (Fig. 4.16).

Each protein has its own specific number and sequence of amino acids. Change the position of an amino acid in a chain and a new protein with different structure and function will be formed. In sickle cell anaemia the haemoglobin differs only slightly from normal haemoglobin in that the amino acid valine replaces glutamic acid as the 6th amino acid in the β globin chains (Fig. 4.17). This changes the shape of the red blood cell to the characteristic sickle shape and reduces its ability to carry oxygen.

Activity

Making proteins from amino acids is similar to playing a game of cards. Each time you shuffle and deal the cards you get a different hand. Imagine you have four amino acids ♣♦♥♠, work out how many different proteins you could make from these four suits. Hint, start by using the same amino acid, e.g. ♣♣♣♣ and ♥♥♥♥, etc.

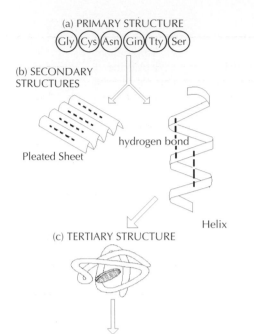

(a) PRIMARY STRUCTURE
(Gly)(Cys)(Asn)(Gin)(Tty)(Ser)

(b) SECONDARY STRUCTURES

Pleated Sheet

hydrogen bond

Helix

(c) TERTIARY STRUCTURE

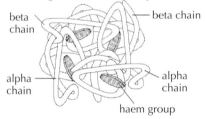

(d) QUATERNARY STRUCTURE of haemoglobin showing the 4 sub-units: 2 alpha and 2 beta chains.

beta chain — beta chain

alpha chain — alpha chain

haem group

Fig. 4.17 Structure of proteins

Structure of proteins

Within proteins several different levels of structure are seen. The primary structure is the order of the amino acids in the chain. The secondary structure results from hydrogen bonding in the chain. The most common type of secondary structure is a helix, e.g. hair. Here hydrogen bonds hold different parts of the same chain together giving flexibility and elasticity to the structure. In the less common pleated sheet structure, hydrogen bonds hold different chains side by side, so the structure is flexible but not elastic, e.g. silk. The tertiary structure results

from folding of the chains. This gives the protein its unique shape and enables it to act in a specific way, e.g. enzymes. Some proteins have a quaternary structure this is where two or more polypeptide chains are arranged into a multisubunit protein, e.g. haemoglobin has four subunits (two beta, β, and two alpha, α) (Fig. 4.17).

The structure of proteins reflects their biological function. Proteins are also classified according to their shape as either globular or fibrous. Fibrous proteins have a structural role and consist of long chains of entwined amino acids, like strands of a rope, e.g. collagen or keratin. Globular proteins have a functional role rather than a structural role and can be compared to a ball of string, e.g. haemoglobin and enzymes. The roles of these proteins are summarised in Table 4.2.

Enzymes

Enzymes are biological catalysts. Catalysts speed up the rate of reaction but are not used up or changed in the reaction. Some enzymes are just pure proteins, others consist of two parts – a protein portion (apoenzyme) and a cofactor. Cofactors can be metals such as iron or organic molecules such as vitamins (these are called coenzyme). The absence of coenzymes can lead to a variety of diseases, e.g. absence of folic acid gives megaloblastic anaemia, absence of thiamin (B_1) leads to beriberi. Enzymes are named after the reaction they catalyse and end in -ase e.g. amylase.

Properties of enzymes

- Enzymes are specific and generally only catalyse one type of chemical reaction. The substance to which the enzyme binds and acts on is called the substrate. Substrates bind to specific sites on the enzyme surface called active sites.
- Enzymes work best at an optimum temperature, this is 37 °C in the body. Low

Table 4.2 Proteins in the body

Structure	Function	Protein
Fibrous	Movement	Actin and myosin are both contractile proteins found in muscle cells
	Structural	Collagen found in ligaments, bones and tendons is the most abundant protein in the body
		Keratin – water proofing protein found in hair and nails
		Elastin – gives elasticity, ligaments and blood vessels
Globular	Catalyst	Increases the rate of chemical reactions in the body, e.g. the enzyme pepsin involved in the digestion of proteins
	Transport	Haemoglobin carries oxygen, lipoproteins carry cholesterol, transferrin carries iron and albumin carries fatty acids
	Buffers	Haemoglobin and plasma proteins, e.g. albumin
	Metabolism	Hormones – regulate growth and metabolic activity, e.g. growth hormone or insulin for the regulation of blood glucose
	Protective	Antibodies (immunoglobulins) help to remove invading bacteria and viruses. Fibrinogen seals wounds

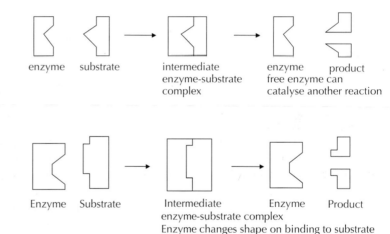

enzyme   substrate   intermediate   enzyme   product
                           enzyme-substrate   free enzyme can
                           complex   catalyse another reaction

Fig. 4.18 Lock and key mechanism.

Enzyme   Substrate   Intermediate   Enzyme   Product
                           enzyme-substrate complex
                           Enzyme changes shape on binding to substrate

Fig. 4.19 Induced fit hypothesis.

temperatures slow reactions down. High temperatures can denature the enzyme by breaking the hydrogen bonds within the enzyme so that the enzyme will no longer work.

- Enzymes work best at an optimum pH, this varies depending on the enzyme. Extremes of pH can denature the enzyme.
- Enzymes can be inhibited – poisons can occupy the 'space' normally filled by the substrate.

Mechanism of enzyme activity

In the lock and key mechanism (Fig. 4.18) the enzyme has a rigid structure. This mechanism has been modified since it is now known that enzymes are flexible and can alter their shape slightly. This new model is known as 'induced fit hypothesis' (Fig. 4.19).

One of the most common genetic disorders is phenylketonuria (PKU). PKU is caused by the lack of the enzyme phenylalanine hydroxylase.

This is because the body is unable to use the amino acid phenylalanine which is present in all foods containing protein. Phenylalanine accumulates in the body resulting in mental retardation. All newborns are tested for PKU by using a blood test called the Guthrie test.

Enzymes are used diagnostically in medicine. Enzymes only react with specific substrates in the sample and they can detect very low concentrations of substrate. The enzyme glucose oxidase is used to test specifically for glucose in blood and urine.

Specific enzyme activity can indicate recent events in the body. After a myocardial infarction (heart attack) the levels of three enzymes, lactate dehydrogenase (LDH), aspartate transaminase (AST) and creatinine kinase (CK) are measured. These enzymes are present in the muscle tissue of the heart and when the tissue is damaged they are released into the blood. The changes in enzyme levels occur over 7 to 9 days and a series of measurements are taken.

Nucleic acids

Nucleic acids are the biggest molecules found in the body. Nucleic acids were first isolated by the Swiss biochemist Miescher from the nuclei of cells, hence their name. There are two types:

- deoxyribonucleic acid (DNA) – makes up the genetic material (chromosomes) and provides instruction for protein synthesis
- ribonucleic acid (RNA) – required for protein synthesis.

Nucleic acids are polymers and their building blocks are nucleotides (Fig. 4.20). Each nucleotide consists of three parts:

- a phosphate group
- a five-carbon sugar
- and a nitrogen-containing base.

The chain of nucleotides in the nucleic acid molecule are linked together through their sugar/phosphate groups (phosphodiester bonds) (Fig. 4.21). There are four different bases in DNA: adenine (A), cytosine (C), thymine (T) and guanine (G). Adenine can only hydrogen-bond with thymine and cytosine with guanine this is called base-pairing. RNA contains uracil (U) instead of thymine (Table 4.3). The sequence of these base pairs determines the genetic makeup of all living things on earth, including you!

The structure of DNA was solved by Crick and Watson in 1953. It is a double helix that can be compared to a spiral staircase (Fig. 4.22). The sugar/phosphate groups provide the handrail or back bone of the staircase and the hydrogen-bonded bases the rungs.

Exercise 4.2

The bases in a strand of DNA are in the order

                        TAACGATGC

What will the order of bases be on the other strand of DNA?

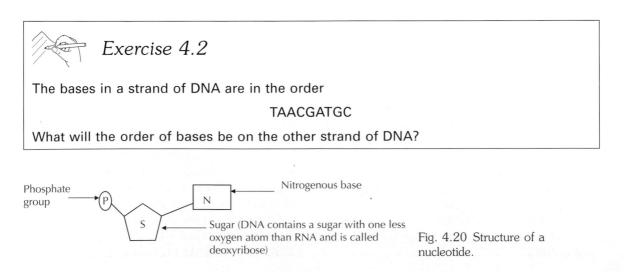

Phosphate group → P

S

Nitrogenous base → N

Sugar (DNA contains a sugar with one less oxygen atom than RNA and is called deoxyribose)

Fig. 4.20 Structure of a nucleotide.

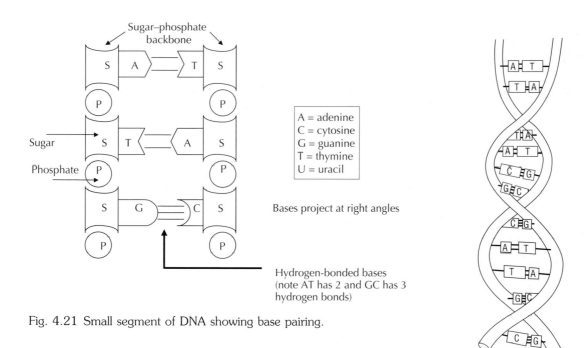

Sugar–phosphate backbone
S
A
T
S
P
P
Sugar
S
T
A
S
Phosphate
P
P
S
G
C
S
P
P
A = adenine
C = cytosine
G = guanine
T = thymine
U = uracil
Bases project at right angles
Hydrogen-bonded bases (note AT has 2 and GC has 3 hydrogen bonds)

Fig. 4.21 Small segment of DNA showing base pairing.

Fig. 4.22 Structure of DNA.

Table 4.3 Some differences between DNA and RNA

	DNA	RNA
Position in cell	Mostly in nucleus but some in mitochondria	Synthesised in nucleus. Messenger RNA (mRNA) is found in the nucleus, transfer RNA(tRNA) is found in the cytoplasm, and ribosomal RNA(rRNA) is found in ribosomes
Function	Forms the genetic material. Provides instructions for protein synthesis. Replicates itself before cell division	Protein synthesis Genetic material in some viruses
Sugar	Deoxyribose	Ribose
Base	Adenine (A) Guanine (G) Cytosine (C) Thymine (T)	Adenine Guanine Cytosine Uracil (U)
Size (relative formula mass)	Very large – thousands of millions	Small, 20 000–40 000
Structure	Double strand, twisted into double helix	Single strand helix

---

⚥ *Activity*

Look at the diagram of the digestive system (Fig. 4.23). Familiarise yourself with all the different parts. What are their functions? Do you know what villi and microvilli are? If not, read a chapter on digestion in a physiology book.

■ ■ Digestion and absorption of biomolecules

In digestion large molecules are broken down in the presence of enzymes to smaller molecules so they can be absorbed. Proteins are digested to amino acids, carbohydrates to monosaccharides and fats to fatty acids and glycerol.

■ Carbohydrates

The digestion of starch starts in the mouth. Salivary amylase in saliva splits starch into dextrins and maltose. The longer food is chewed the more effective the enzymes.

Most carbohydrate digestion takes place within the small intestine. The pancreas secretes pancreatic amylase into the duodenum of the small intestine and this hydrolyses any starch left into mainly maltose. The enzymes of the brush border then complete digestion.

Each day about 500 g of monosaccharides (depending on diet) are absorbed into the blood capillaries of the intestine (ileum) (Fig. 4.24).

Lactose intolerance is caused by the lack of the enzyme lactase. Milk is the main source of lactose in the diet. Lactase is secreted by all babies but deficiency in adults is very common. The undigested lactose remains in the lumen of small intestine causing diarrhoea and abdomi-

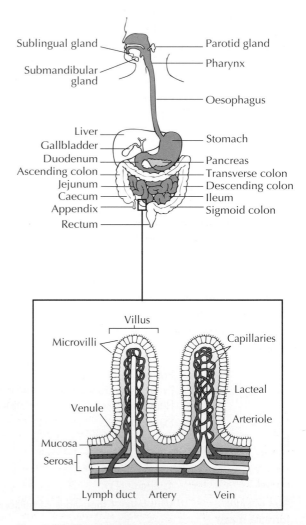

Fig. 4.23 The digestive system.

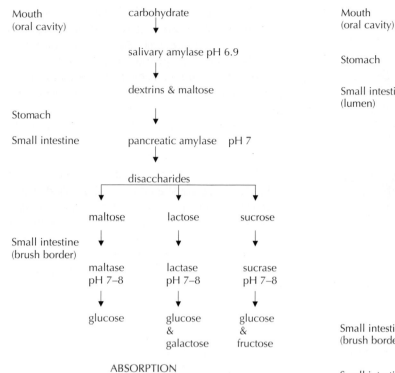

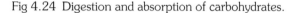

ABSORPTION
All the sugars are absorbed into the blood capillaries of the intestine and transported to the liver via the hepatic portal system

Fig 4.24 Digestion and absorption of carbohydrates.

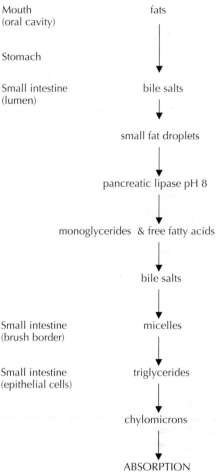

ABSORPTION
Absorbed via the central lacteals of the villi into the lymph system. The lymph drains into the thoracic duct which empties into the left subclavian vein in the base of the neck. Lipids are then transported to the liver via the circulatory system

Fig. 4.25 Digestion and absorption of fat.

nal bloating and pain. The treatment for lactose intolerance is either to follow a lactose-free diet or to add commercially available lactase enzyme to milk.

Fats (lipids)

Fat digestion only occurs in the small intestine (Fig. 4.25). Fat and its digestion products are insoluble in water, forming large globules in the intestine. The enzyme lipase is unable to digest these large globules. To overcome this problem bile is secreted from the liver into the duodenum. Bile is a watery mixture of ions, bile salts, bile pigments, cholesterol, lecithin and mucus. The bile salts emulsify the fats, that is, they break down the fat globules into smaller droplets. Lipase then digests the fat into free fatty acids and monoglycerides (one fatty acid chain).

The hydrophobic ends of the bile salts cling to the fat globule, whilst the negative polar ends

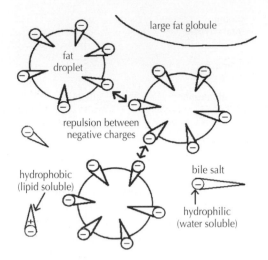

Fig. 4.26 Formation of an emulsion.

dissolve in the water. This pulls small fat droplets off the larger globule. The negative charges on the polar ends of these drops repel other drops and this stabilises the emulsion (Fig. 4.26).

Bile salts are also needed for the absorption of the insoluble digestion products monoglycerides and fatty acids. As soon as they are formed they are combined with lecithin and

cholesterol to form micelles. This allows rapid absorption of fat and fat soluble vitamins into the cells lining the villi. About 80 g of fat is absorbed each day in the small intestine.

Once inside the cells of the intestinal epithelium the free fatty acids and monoglycerides are reassembled to triglycerides. They become coated with a layer of lipoprotein, cholesterol and phospholipids to form chylomicrons. The chylomicrons are too large to enter the blood capillaries so enter the central lacteals of the villi. The milky substance formed is called chyle. The lacteals are part of the lymphatic system.

When there are insufficient bile salts in the bile or if the bile becomes too concentrated the cholesterol it contains starts to crystallise out to form gallstones. These sharp gallstones cause pain when the gallbladder or its duct contracts. Gallstones often pass out of the gallbladder and lodge in the hepatic and common bile ducts, this prevents the flow of bile into the duodenum and results in obstructive jaundice which is characterised by yellow colouration of the skin. Gallstones are easily diagnosed by using ultrasound and are generally treated by non-invasive techniques such as drugs to dissolve the stones or shock waves to break the stones up (lithotripsy).

Activity

How could you use the above information to explain to a patient suffering from gallstones why the pain is increased when they eat fatty food, why their faeces are fatty, smelly and float, and why they might be slightly jaundiced?

Proteins

Protein digestion starts in the stomach (Fig. 4.27). The enzyme pepsin responsible for protein digestion is secreted in its inactive form pepsinogen. The acid conditions of the stomach convert pepsinogen to pepsin. Pepsin digests proteins into polypeptides. Protein digestion continues in the duodenum. The pancreatic enzymes – trypsin, chymotrypsin and car-

boxypeptidase are all secreted in their inactive form.

The enzyme enterokinase converts trypsinogen to trypsin. Trypsin then converts all the other enzymes to their active form. They digest polypeptides, forming peptides. The brush border enzymes carboxypeptidase, aminopeptidase and dipeptidase act on peptides and dipeptides breaking off individual amino acids. 50 g of amino acids need to be absorbed each day

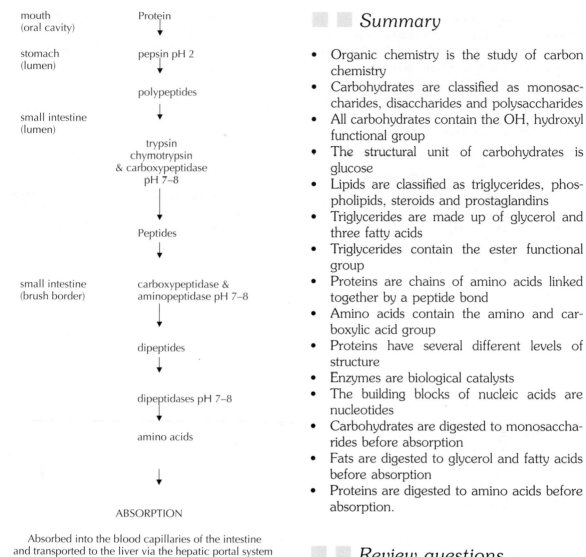

mouth
(oral cavity)

Protein

stomach
(lumen)

pepsin pH 2

polypeptides

small intestine
(lumen)

trypsin
chymotrypsin
& carboxypeptidase
pH 7–8

Peptides

small intestine
(brush border)

carboxypeptidase &
aminopeptidase pH 7–8

dipeptides

dipeptidases pH 7–8

amino acids

ABSORPTION

Absorbed into the blood capillaries of the intestine
and transported to the liver via the hepatic portal system

Fig. 4.27 Digestion and absorption of proteins.

to obtain a positive nitrogen balance – that is, intake of protein (nitrogen) synthesis exceeds the rate of breakdown and loss. In negative nitrogen balance, protein breakdown exceeds protein synthesis, this can occur during illness, e.g. infection or burns. The amino acids are then absorbed into the blood capillaries of the intestines.

Summary

- Organic chemistry is the study of carbon chemistry
- Carbohydrates are classified as monosaccharides, disaccharides and polysaccharides
- All carbohydrates contain the OH, hydroxyl functional group
- The structural unit of carbohydrates is glucose
- Lipids are classified as triglycerides, phospholipids, steroids and prostaglandins
- Triglycerides are made up of glycerol and three fatty acids
- Triglycerides contain the ester functional group
- Proteins are chains of amino acids linked together by a peptide bond
- Amino acids contain the amino and carboxylic acid group
- Proteins have several different levels of structure
- Enzymes are biological catalysts
- The building blocks of nucleic acids are nucleotides
- Carbohydrates are digested to monosaccharides before absorption
- Fats are digested to glycerol and fatty acids before absorption
- Proteins are digested to amino acids before absorption.

Review questions

4.1.   The structure of aspirin is shown (Fig. 4.28). Identify the carboxylic acid functional group.

4.2.   Why are the enzymes involved in protein digestion secreted in their inactive form?

4.3.   People who suffer from lactose intolerance cannot drink milk. However they can eat cheese and yoghurt, why?

4.4.   Why must patients inject hormones such as growth hormone and insulin rather than taking them orally?

4.5.   Clinistix® tests for glucose in urine. The conditions for storage of Clinistix® are: room temperature (15 to 30 °C), not in direct sunlight, away from moisture and the contents should be discarded within 6 months of opening. What effect would the following conditions have on test results of the Clinistix®?

a) Storing the Clinistix® in the fridge

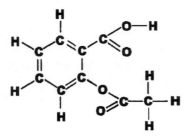

Fig 4.28 Aspirin.

b) Storing the Clinistix® at a temperature above 50 °C
c) Using Clinistix® after the expiry date.

Further reading

Marieb, E.N. (2000). *Human Anatomy and Physiology* (5th edn). Benjamin Cummings, Redwood City, California.

Watson, R. (ed). (1999). *Essential Science for Nursing Students. An Introductory Test.* Baillière Tindall, London.

Sackhein, G.I. & Lehman, D.D. (1998). *Chemistry for the Health Sciences* (8th edn). Prentice Hall, London.

British Nutrition Foundation. Homepage: http://www.nutrition.org.uk/Facts/energynut/carbo.html

Chapter Five
CELLS

Learning objectives

By the end of the chapter the reader will be able to:
- Explain that all organisms are made from cells
- Explain the differences between cells, viruses and prions
- Describe the structure of human cells
- Describe mitosis and meiosis
- Link abnormal cell structure and growth to disease.

Introduction

Cells are the basic unit of life and yet they cannot be seen easily without a microscope because they are so small (human cells are about 25 micrometres (µm) wide). As a nurse, you could be taking samples of cells, e.g. blood, biopsies, throat swabs from patients for analysis in the laboratory. The tests might be simply counting and sorting the cells into different types but this can tell us a lot about the well-being of a patient and how to treat them, e.g. a low red blood cell count could indicate anaemia. The human body contains 60 billion (6×10^{13}) cells and about two hundred different cell types; fortunately they all share the same basic structure.

Two cell types

There are two main types of cells – eukaryotic cells (animal, plant and fungi) and prokaryotic cells (bacteria). Eukaryotic cells have their genetic material, deoxyribonucleic acid (DNA), packaged into chromosomes within a nucleus. Prokaryotic cells – bacteria – are about 1 micrometre (µm) in diameter whereas eukaryotic cells can be as much as 200 µm in diameter. These much smaller cells have their DNA free in the cell cytoplasm. Despite these differences, we can think of both human and bacterial cells as genetic material surrounded by cytoplasm which is enclosed by a thin membrane (Fig. 5.1).

Eukaryotic cells interact with each other

All complex organisms are made from cells in much the same way as a house is built from bricks. The cells are organised and interact to perform different functions; those that carry out the same function are grouped together to form a tissue, e.g. liver tissue is made from liver cells. Different tissues are grouped together to form organs, e.g. the heart is made from muscle and nervous tissue which work together so that the heart pumps blood round the body.

For activities carried out by the body, organs are grouped in systems. Urine production and excretion involves the kidneys, ureters, bladder and urethra, collectively called the urinary or excretory system. The organ systems are packaged together to form multicellular organisms, e.g. humans, animals, plants and fungi. It is amazing that such complexity can be derived from a single basic structure.

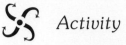

Activity

Put some Sellotape on the back of your hand and peel it off. Hold the tape to the light and see the outer skin cells.

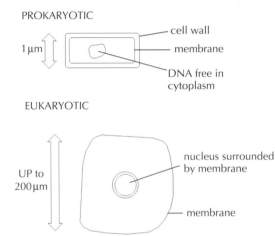

Fig. 5.1 Eukaryotic and prokaryotic cell structure.

Prokaryotic cells are unicellular

Prokaryotic cells (bacteria) are not organised into structures like human cells. One bacterium is a single cell (unicellular) capable of independent life. Hundreds of different kinds live on you! Until recently it was not thought that different types of bacteria could interact together in an organised way. Now it seems that some bacteria can group together to form biofilms which cause disease in the lungs, gums, ears and kidneys. The bottom cells of the biofilm stick to the tissue surface whereas the outer cells secrete a slimy coating which protects them from antibiotics and being attacked by white blood cells. Bacteria working together like this is a bit like an organ system; different types carry out different functions for their mutual benefit so that all of them can survive in hostile environments.

Viruses and Prions

Viruses and prions are not cells. They can be thought of as being somewhere between the living and the dead! However they depend on cells for their replication. Nearly all of them are smaller than the smallest cell (Table 5.1).

Viruses have either ribonucleic acid (RNA) or deoxyribonucleic acid (DNA) as their genetic material; they can survive outside their host cell in an extracellular state. In the extracellular state, a protein coat and sometimes a membranous envelope surrounds the genetic material. In this state they are called virus particles or virions.

Prions are made entirely from glycoproteins and have no nucleic acids. Like viruses they have an extracellular state but little is known about prions.

When cells are infected with a virus or prion, it is usually damaging to the health of the infected organism, e.g. influenza and mad cow

Activity

Look at a bacterial biofilm by scraping some plaque from your teeth. If you can, look at it under a microscope.
You can also see the biofilm by using disclosing tablets on your teeth.

Table 5.1 Differences between cells, viruses and prions

Structure	Genetic material	Width (μm)
Eukaryotic cell, e.g. red blood cell, muscle cell	DNA	7–200
Prokaryotic cell, e.g. *Pseudomonas aeruginosa*, *Streptococcus pneumoniae*	DNA	0.3–50
Viruses, e.g. influenza virus	RNA or DNA	0.02–0.3
Prions e.g. bovine spongiform encephalopathy prion (BSE)	None	0.0002–0.002

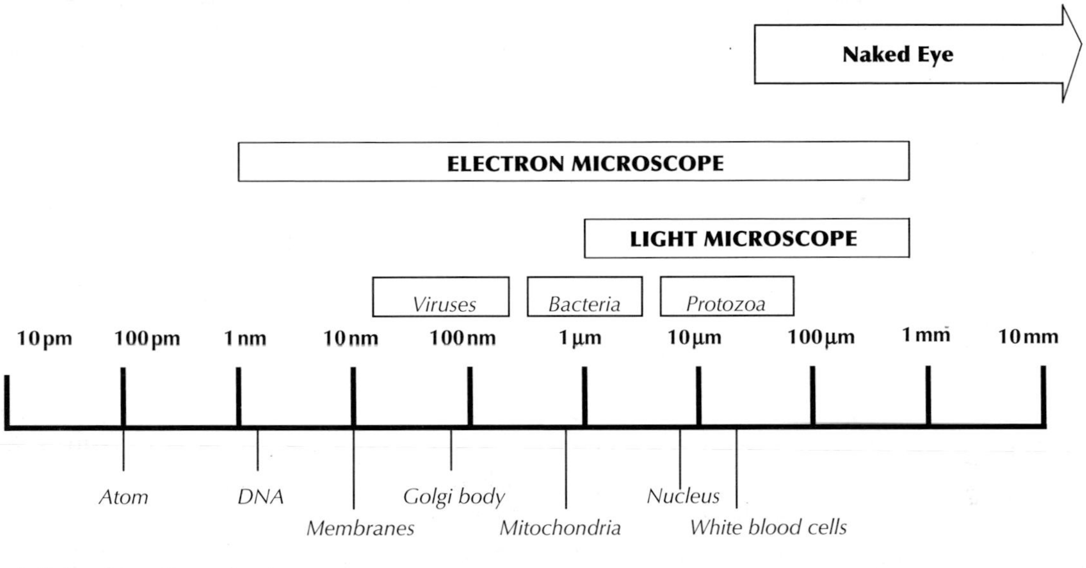

Fig. 5.2 Looking through microscopes.

Activity

Make a list of as many human cells as you can. Do you think they will all look the same? Find a picture of them in a text book and see if their structure reflects their function.

---

disease (Creutzfeldt-Jakob syndrome) caused by a virus and a prion respectively.

Cell structure

The small size of cells means that the detailed structure of cells and viruses can only be seen with an electron microscope which can magnify objects about 100 000 times. An electron microscope can be used diagnostically, e.g. examination of infant faecal samples for human rotavirus.

Electron microscopes are very big and expensive and not usually found in a basic hospital laboratory. Fortunately, microscopes that use

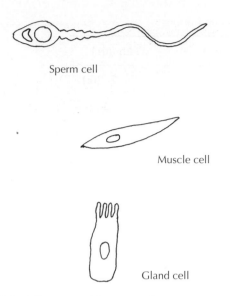

Sperm cell

Muscle cell

Gland cell

Fig. 5.3 Differentiated human cells.

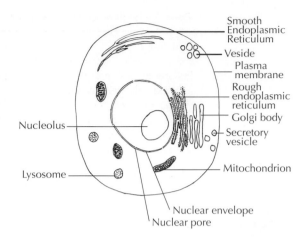

Fig. 5.4 Human cell structure.

visible light to illuminate specimens are cheaper and widely available. Light microscopes, which magnify objects by 1000, let you see some internal structures of eukaryotic cells like the nucleus and their shape but not much more than the shape of prokaryotic cells (Fig. 5.2).

Although eukaryotic cells share the same fundamental structure, they can be differentiated from each other. For example, cells lining the respiratory tract are ciliated to help in the removal of mucus and do not look the same as a sperm cell which is the only motile human cell (Fig. 5.3). The differences reflect the specific function of the cell, but remember that they all originated from a single, fertilised egg. Interestingly, cancer cells dedifferentiate, they are rounder than the original cells and the cell membrane is more permeable, which allows more fluids into them.

Human cell structure

Each cell has an outer cytoplasmic or plasma membrane, which encloses the jelly-like cytoplasm and genetic material in a nucleus. In the cytoplasm there are many organelles, each of which has a specific function and secretory

vesicles (Fig. 5.4). Membranes surround the organelles, which keeps them separate from each other and allows them to operate under different conditions. Separation of the organelles is very important; if they had no surrounding membrane to retain their structures the cell would die. Nevertheless organelles can communicate with each other via special pores in their membranes to carry out complex functions like secretion.

Membrane structure

The importance of membranes is clear but what exactly is a membrane and what does it do? Basically, it separates two solutions, i.e. the membrane around the cell separates it from the fluids inside and outside the cell. The basic structure of membranes is the same in all cells. They are made mainly from a group of molecules called phospholipids and proteins. Two layers of phospholipids form a hydrophobic (water hating) bilayer or barrier because of their chemical structure. The proteins are inserted into the bilayer and are important for the functions of the membranes, e.g. they form pores or channels through the membrane to form a transport system for molecules or act as receptor molecules (Fig. 5.5).

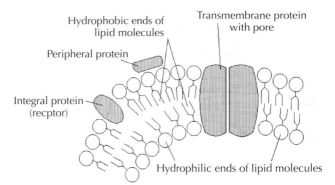

Fig. 5.5 The molecular composition of a cell membrane.

 Activity

You can make a lipid bilayer in water simply by dropping some drops of oil into water. They will not disperse but will form a ball showing the hydrophobicity of the phospholipids.

Although the structure in Fig. 5.5 might make you think that the structure is fixed, the molecules move about, they are not a solid layer like butter or margarine. For this reason membranes are often referred to as fluid membranes. This fluidity aids the transport of molecules within and between organelles.

Movement of large molecules

The structure of membranes also allows the movement of large molecules through them by exocytosis, endocytosis and phagocytosis. They all rely on membrane fusion. Membranes do not normally fuse together, if they did all the organelles within a cell would fuse together with catastrophic effects for the cell. The fusion of membranes is inhibited by the high negative surface charge of the phosphate groups on the phospholipids and the fact that there are no free edges on membranes.

Exocytosis

Exocytosis is the fusion of an internal vesicle with the plasma membrane so that the vesicle contents are expelled from the cell. For example secretory proteins are enclosed by a membrane from the Golgi body. The secretory vesicle is transported to the plasma membrane where the protein is released into the extracellular space.

Enveloped viruses (viruses surrounded by a membrane derived from the host cell), e.g. human immunodeficiency virus (HIV), influenza virus, infect a host cell by effectively reversing exocytosis. The virus enters the cell by fusing with the plasma membrane and releasing the genetic material from the virus into the cell cytoplasm where it replicates (Fig. 5.6).

Endocytosis

Endocytosis is the process when only a small region of the plasma membrane folds inwards or is invaginated to form a vesicle about $1\,\mu m$ in diameter. Small volumes of extracellular fluid enter the cell in this way, this is sometimes called cell drinking or pinocytosis.

Phagocytosis

Phagocytosis is the intake of large particles such as bacteria or cell debris, e.g. dead red

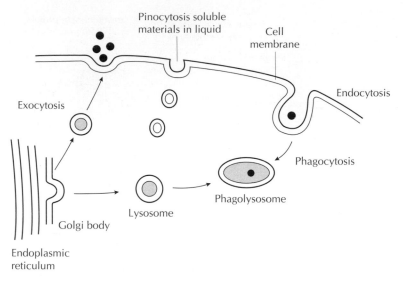

Fig. 5.6 Exocytosis, endocytosis and phagocytosis.

Table 5.2 Human cell organelles

Organelle	Function
Nucleus	Isolates DNA from the cell
Ribosomes	Provide the site for protein synthesis
Endoplasmic reticulum (rough, ribosomes attached; smooth, no ribosomes attached)	Protein modification (rough), lipid synthesis (smooth)
Golgi bodies	Final protein structure changes; sugars synthesised and attached to proteins (glycoproteins) or lipids (glycolipids) or linked to form starches; secretion, storage
Vesicles	Storage and transport of molecules
Mitochondria	Energy (ATP) production
Lysosomes	Breakdown of cell debris in an acid environment
Peroxisomes	Bile acids synthesis, detoxification of molecules

blood cells (erythrocytes). The unwanted particle is bound to the membrane of the cell; the membrane expands and then engulfs it by forming a large vesicle. In the human macrophage, a special kind of white blood cell, large vesicles of at least 1–2 μm diameter and sometimes larger are seen. The vesicles usually fuse with lysosomes to destroy unwanted particles. Around 10^{11} dead red blood cells are destroyed every day by macrophages in this way.

Human cell organelles

Human cell organelles are membrane bound except the ribosomes, their functions are shown in Table 5.2.

The nucleus

The nucleus is the largest organelle and is often called the brain of the cell because it controls

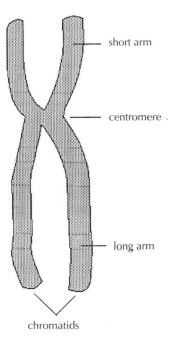

Fig. 5.7 Structure of a chromosome.

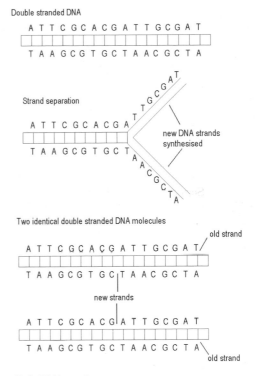

Fig. 5.8 DNA replication.

what the cell does. A double membrane, the nuclear envelope, surrounds it. The nucleus contains the chromosomes – these are long threads of DNA with proteins called histones attached to them. Each chromosome has a centromere, which divides most chromosomes into a short and long arm (Fig. 5.7). The centromere is important for chromosome separation during cell division.

In human cells there are 23 pairs of chromosomes, 46 chromosomes in all. Each pair of chromosomes is homologous, i.e. they are the same in size and shape except for the sex chromosomes where an X and Y chromosome may be a pair in a male and XX in a female. All of the chromosomes together form the human genome for which we now know the complete sequence of the DNA bases on every chromosome. However the identification and function of all the genes is an ongoing task.

DNA replication

At cell division, the DNA in the nucleus is duplicated so that each new cell receives a full set of chromosomes. This is possible because of the double helix structure of DNA. The two long DNA molecules, which make up each chromosome, are attached through their bases adenine, cytosine, guanine and thymine. The attachment is very specific, i.e. adenine will only pair with thymine and guanine will only pair with cytosine. The specificity of the pairing between the bases allows DNA replication or copying to be a highly accurate process and ensures that each cell has the same genetic information. Before DNA can be replicated, the two strands have to be separated, so that a complementary strand can be synthesised. Therefore each new cell receives one old and one new strand of DNA (Fig. 5.8).

After replication, the DNA is folded and twisted with proteins called histones to form

Table 5.3 The genetic code

Codon	Amino acid	Codon	Amino acid	Codon	Amino acid	Codon	Amino acid
UUU	Phenylalanine	CUU	Leucine	GUU	Valine	AUU	Isoleucine
UUC	Phenylalanine	CUC	Leucine	GUC	Valine	AUC	Isoleucine
UUG	Leucine	CUG	Leucine	GUG	Valine	AUG	START (Methionine)
UUA	Leucine	CUA	Leucine	GUA	Valine	AUA	Isoleucine
UCU	Serine	CCU	Proline	GCU	Alanine	ACU	Threonine
UCC	Serine	CCC	Proline	GCC	Alanine	ACC	Threonine
UCG	Serine	CCG	Proline	GCG	Alanine	ACG	Threonine
UCA	Serine	CCA	Proline	GCA	Alanine	ACA	Threonine
UGU	Cysteine	CGU	Arginine	GGU	Glycine	AGU	Serine
UGC	Cysteine	CGC	Arginine	GGC	Glycine	AGC	Serine
UGG	Tryptophan	CGG	Arginine	GGG	Glycine	AGG	Arginine
UGA	STOP	CGA	Arginine	GGA	Glycine	AGA	Arginine
UAU	Tyrosine	CAU	Histidine	GAU	Aspartic	AAU	Asparagine
UAC	Tyrosine	CAC	Histidine	GAC	Aspartic	AAC	Asparagine
UAG	STOP	CAG	Glutamine	GAG	Glutamic	AAG	Lysine
UAA	STOP	CAA	Glutamine	GAA	Glutamic	AAA	Lysine

two sets of condensed chromosomes ready for cell division. These are the structures used to identify the different chromosomes. You may have seen pictures of them used to help patients undergoing genetic counselling.

Nucleolus

In a growing cell there is also a nucleolus where the subunits of ribosomes, needed to synthesise proteins, are made. Molecules can be moved into and out of the nucleus through pore proteins, which go across both membrane bilayers. Receptor proteins on the outer surface trigger the copying of DNA for specific genes into messenger ribonucleic acid (mRNA), which is then transported into the cytoplasm. This process is called transcription.

The genetic code

The complementary, single strand of mRNA contains the same genetic information as DNA but one of the bases, thymine, is replaced by uracil in RNA. The sequence of the bases forms the genetic code. Three bases (one codon) code for one amino acid or a start or stop signal, which allows the translation of the message in DNA into RNA and then amino acids (Table 5.3). Transcription and translation are the two processes required for protein synthesis.

Exercise 5.1

1. What would be the amino acid sequence determined by the codon sequence below?
UUUCAAGUGAACCUG
2. What would be the amino acid sequence if:
   (a) G was removed?
   (b) U was replaced with C?

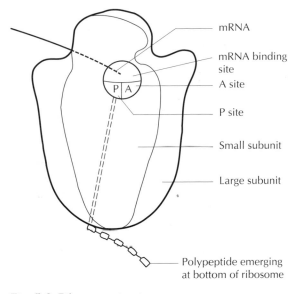

mRNA

mRNA binding site

A site

P site

Small subunit

Large subunit

Polypeptide emerging at bottom of ribosome

Fig. 5.9 Ribosome structure.

Ribosomes

Ribosomes are the site of protein synthesis. They consist of a small and a large subunit and are made from ribosomal RNAs (rRNAs) and proteins. The subunits are free in the cytoplasm and only come together when a protein is synthesised. The small subunit has a binding site for the mRNA formed in the nucleus. The large subunit has two binding sites for transfer RNA (tRNA), an acceptor site (A site) and a peptide site (P site). It also has a membrane binding site and an exit site for the newly emerging protein (Fig. 5.9).

Endoplasmic reticulum

The nuclear envelope, endoplasmic reticulum (ER), Golgi bodies and some vesicles form a continuous membrane system in the cell to provide the correct conditions for the synthesis of cellular molecules. They can be thought of as an assembly line for making proteins.

When mRNA moves out of the nucleus it either becomes associated with ribosomes attached to the endoplasmic reticulum (rough

ER) on the side facing the cytoplasm or with ribosomes free in the cytoplasm. It is here that translation of the mRNA into amino acids takes place. The process requires tRNA molecules. They are often called adaptor molecules because they react with both mRNA by means of an anticodon (a sequence of bases which correspond to those of the codon) and the correct amino acid.

Protein synthesis (translation)

Proteins are synthesised from amino acids which are synthesised by a process called translation. The sequence of amino acids in proteins is determined by the codons in mRNA. Just one altered codon can make an entirely different protein.

The first codon, the start codon, interacts with a special start tRNA, with its amino acid attached in the P site of the ribosome. The next codon in the sequence interacts with its correct tRNA and binds to the A site. A peptide bond is formed between the two amino acids and the bond between the start tRNA and its amino acid is broken to release the tRNA. This moves the tRNA in the A-site to the P site and aligns the next codon to be read in the A site for attachment to a new tRNA. In this way the mRNA is read to form a growing polypeptide chain (elongation) until a stop codon is reached and protein synthesis ends (termination) (see Fig. 5.10).

Endoplasmic reticulum (ER)

Proteins do not stay as a long linear shape – they have to be folded into a three-dimensional shape to function properly. This takes place in the rough ER. Incorrectly folded proteins are detected in the ER and expelled for breakdown (degradation).

The ER close to the nucleus is tightly stacked (Fig. 5.11) but as it gets further away the folds become looser and the tube wider with fewer or no ribosomes attached. This is the smooth ER where lipids are synthesised and added to

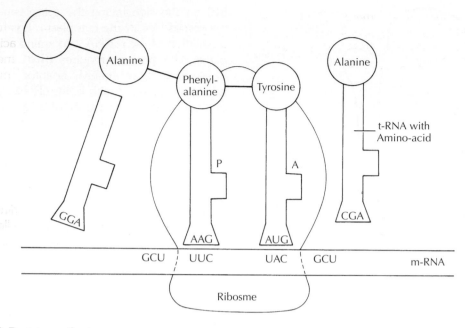

Fig. 5.10 Protein synthesis.

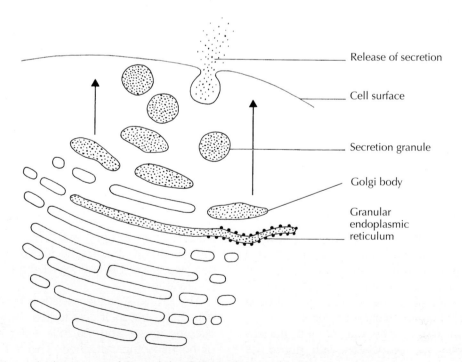

Fig. 5.11 The endoplasmic reticulum and the Golgi body assembly line.

the proteins made in the rough ER. Towards the cell membrane the tubes become narrower again ending in vesicles, which are pinched off for transport to the Golgi body.

Golgi body

The Golgi body is a series of flattened membranes. It changes the proteins, which enter it, so that they carry out a specific function. Vesicles from the ER fuse in one region of the Golgi body, are modified and transported to another region and then released as a vesicle. The vesicle can either fuse immediately with the plasma membrane (exocytosis) and release its content or be stored until another signal is received, e.g. a hormone before it is released.

Lysosomes

Lysosomes are simply vesicles, which are pinched off either from the ER or the Golgi body. In humans they contain around 40 enzymes that break down toxic components, for this reason large numbers are seen in liver cells. The enzymes only function at low pH. If lysosomes are disrupted then the contents destroy the cellular components which are close to them. Lysosomes are also responsible for degrading unwanted or old cellular components. Defective lysosomal enzymes cause lysosome storage diseases of which Tay-Sachs disease is a well documented example.

Peroxisomes

Peroxisomes are found in high numbers in liver and kidney cells. They are small membrane-bound organelles that contain enzymes which degrade fatty acids and amino acids and synthesise bile acids. Hydrogen peroxide (also used as hair bleach) is formed during the degradation process. This is very toxic to cells but peroxisomes have a special enzyme called catalase, which degrades the hydrogen peroxide to water and oxygen.

Mitochondria

All of the reactions in the cell need energy, which is produced in the mitochondria. The number of mitochondria in the cell depends on its activity, for example liver cells will contain about 1000 mitochondria, muscle cells many more but yeast cells only two. Mitochondria have two membranes. One is an inner, tightly folded membrane that contains the enzymes, which make a chemical form of energy, adenosine triphosphate (ATP), from the breakdown products of digestion. The other, an outer membrane, has pores large enough to allow ATP to be released into the cell to drive all of the different activities of the cell.

Mitochondria also contain DNA, which is inherited but only from the mother. A distinct group of diseases caused by defective mitochondria are recognised in humans often resulting in fatigue and/or muscle weakness.

The cytoskeleton

We have already seen that cells have a definite shape. The jelly-like cytoplasm alone cannot maintain a fixed shape so how is this achieved? Just beneath the cell membrane is an internal skeleton or cytoskeleton made of protein rods called actin and tubules called microtubules. This, together with the plasma membrane and the extracellular matrix (mixture of glycoproteins and proteins on the outside surface of the cell), gives the cell its characteristic shape. Any breakdown in the links is potentially lethal; muscular dystrophy is just one example.

The extracellular matrix also helps cells to recognise each other and distinguish foreign bodies. This is very important for the function of the immune system and helps to explain why it is important to match organs for transplant or blood for transfusions.

Several microtubules can form cylinders called centrioles from which cilia and flagella arise. The centrioles remain as the basal body of the flagella or cilia. Many of our cells are ciliated e.g. those

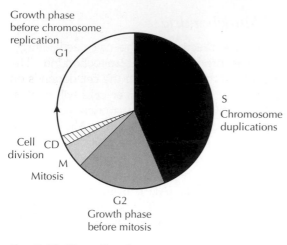

Growth phase
before chromosome
replication
G1

S
Chromosome
duplications

Cell CD
division
M
Mitosis

G2
Growth phase
before mitosis

Fig. 5.12 The cell cycle.

lining the respiratory tract, flagellated cells are associated with free movement. In humans, the only example is the sperm cell.

Growth of cells and cell division

The number of cells in the human body is regulated by cell division and cell death. All human cells except testicular and ovarian cells, divide to increase their number by a process called mitosis, e.g. during growth, for the repair of skin tissue damage to replace old, dead cells. Cell death decreases cell number and occurs either by apoptosis or necrosis. Apoptosis removes unwanted cells throughout life and is especially important in fetal development. Necrosis is the destruction of damaged cells accompanied by inflammation, e.g. in gangrene.

The cell cycle and mitosis

Cell growth and division are described in a regular series of events called the cell cycle (Fig. 5.12).

The length of each stage of the cycle varies with the type of cell. Most of the time before cell division is spent in interphase, the period of

Table 5.4 Cell cycle times of specialised cells

Type of cell	Cell cycle
Bone marrow	10–18 hours
Egg and sperm	2–3 days
Neutrophils (white blood cells)	13 days
Red blood cells	120 days
Mature nerve cells of the central nervous system	Lifetime of body

growth before DNA is replicated. Mature nerve cells are permanently in interphase because they do not divide. Mitosis or division phase is a small part of the whole cycle and occurs in about one-tenth of your cells every day. The average cell cycle time for some cells is shown in Table 5.4.

Three stages are recognised in interphase:

1. Primary growth (G1) when cytoplasmic components are synthesised.
2. Synthesis (S1) when DNA is replicated.
3. A second, shorter growth phase (G2) when the proteins needed for mitosis are synthesised.

Four distinct phases of mitosis are recognised (Fig. 5.13):

- Prophase where the chromosomes that were replicated in interphase condense (become shorter and thicker by the DNA coiling tightly) to become two chromatids joined at the centromere. Microtubles are made for spindle assembly and enter the nuclear region as the nuclear membrane and cytoskeleton break down and the nucleolus disappears.
- Metaphase where the chromosomes attach to the spindle at their centromeres (point of joining of the two identical chromosomes) and line up at the centre of the cell.
- Anaphase where the chromosomes are pulled apart at the centromere and one set moves to each new cell. The movement is brought about by the shortening and lengthening of the microtubules forming the spindle.

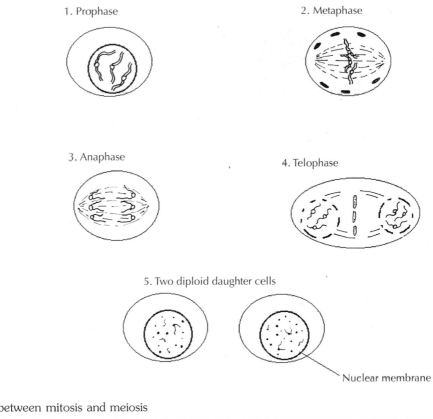

1. Prophase

2. Metaphase

3. Anaphase

4. Telophase

5. Two diploid daughter cells

Nuclear membrane

Fig. 5.13 Mitosis.

Table 5.5 The differences between mitosis and meiosis

Properties	Mitosis	Meiosis
Number of nuclear divisions	One	Two
Total number of cells on completion	Two	Four
Chromosome number (n)	2n the same number as the parent cell (human 46)	1n half the number of the parent cell (human 23)
Type of cells	Body (somatic) cells	Testicular and ovarian (germ) cells
Occurrence in humans	Throughout life	After puberty
Function	Cell maintenance and repair, growth; produces genetically identical cells	Production of sperm and eggs; allows gene recombination

- Telophase where a complete set of chromosomes is at each end of the cell, the spindle falls apart, the nuclear membrane reforms and two nucleoli are visible.

Finally the two cells separate (cytokinesis). Both cells are the same; each cell has a nucleus with a set of chromosomes from the original cell and a set synthesised during the cell cycle.

Meiosis

Meiosis is a special form of cell division in which the number of parental chromosomes are reduced by half (Fig. 5.14).

In meiosis I or reduction division, one of each pair of chromosomes (23 pairs, 46 chromosomes) is separated into two cells. The differences between mitosis and meiosis are summarised in Table 5.5.

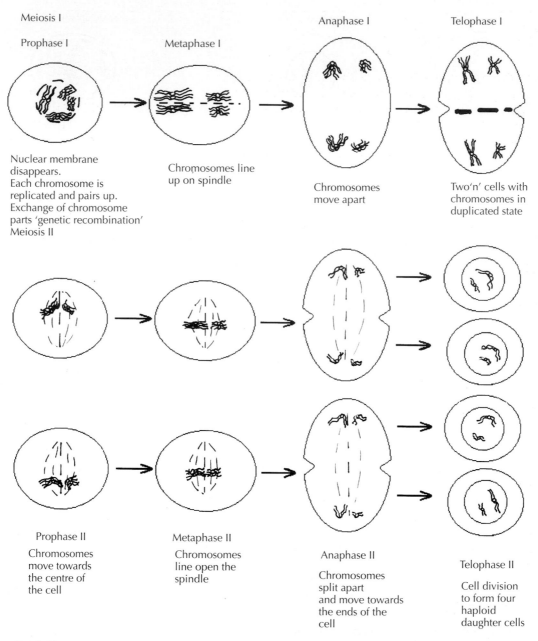

Meiosis I

Prophase I

Nuclear membrane disappears.
Each chromosome is replicated and pairs up.
Exchange of chromosome parts 'genetic recombination'
Meiosis II

Metaphase I

Chromosomes line up on spindle

Anaphase I

Chromosomes move apart

Telophase I

Two 'n' cells with chromosomes in duplicated state

Prophase II
Chromosomes move towards the centre of the cell

Metaphase II
Chromosomes line open the spindle

Anaphase II
Chromosomes split apart and move towards the ends of the cell

Telophase II
Cell division to form four haploid daughter cells

Fig. 5.14 Meiosis.

The stages of this division are:

- Interphase: the dividing cell replicates the DNA of each chromosome so that it becomes two chromatids joined at the centromere as in mitosis (homologous pairs).

- Prophase I: the DNA condenses, again, like mitosis and the chromosomes (four chromatids) become visible. They line up gene by gene and are held together by a mixture of RNA and proteins. The chromatids from each parent break at the same point, swap

Exercise 5.2

Match the definitions (1 to 4) with the terms (a to d):
1. One of the copies of a duplicated chromosome
2. The chromosomes on the spindle pull apart and move to each new cell
3. The separation of two cells
4. Proteins are synthesised but DNA is not replicated

(a) cytokinesis
(b) chromatid
(c) meiosis II
(d) anaphase

bits and reseal them – a process called crossing over. This is literally a mixing up of genes from each original parental chromosome. The number of genes remains the same but they are in different combinations.

- Metaphase I: The chromosomes line up on the spindle.
- Anaphase I: Each homologous chromosome is separated and moves to opposite ends of the spindle.
- Telophase I: Cell division to form two haploid (n) cells with one duplicated chromosome in each.

In the second division meiosis II, proteins are synthesised but DNA is not replicated. Four stages are recognised:

- Prophase II – the chromosomes become visible.
- Metaphase II – the spindle aligns the chromosomes.
- Anaphase II – the centromeres part and each chromatid pair becomes two chromosomes which are pulled to opposite ends of the cell.
- Telophase II – the separated sets of chromosomes are enclosed by a nuclear membrane. This is followed by the cell dividing into two. Four cells are produced with half the original number of chromosomes.

Summary

- All cells are composed of DNA in cytoplasm surrounded by a membrane
- Viruses and prions are not cells

- Human cell function depends on membrane-bound organelles which separates them from each other in the cytoplasm
- Cell number is regulated by cell division and cell death
- Mitosis and meiosis are the processes of division in human cells

Review questions

5.1. Explain the difference between human and bacterial cells.

5.2. Why do membranes need to be 'fluid' structures?

5.3. Distinguish between transcription and translation.

5.4. Explain the difference between exocytosis and endocytosis.

5.5. Name the two processes of nuclear division in human cells. Why are two processes needed?

5.6. Explain why viruses and prions are not cells.

Further reading

Young, B. & Heath, J.W. (2000) *Wheater's Functional Histology* (4th edn). Churchill Livingstone (Harcourt Publishers Ltd), London.
Marieb, E.N. (2000). *Human Anatomy and Physiology* (5th edn). Benjamin Cummings, Redwood City, California.

Chapter Six
GENETICS

Learning objectives

By the end of this chapter the reader will be able to:
- Relate genetic variation to genetic recombination of genes at the same locus
- Distinguish between recessive and dominant genes
- Calculate the probability of inheritance of a single gene disorder
- Describe the significance of multifactorial inheritance
- Recognise the possible role of the nurse in genetic screening and counselling.

Introduction

Genetics is the study of inherited variations and characteristics (traits). Genes are a unique sequence of deoxyribonucleic acid (DNA) which code for a particular protein. Our genes are inherited from our parents – they determine what we look like and how we react to certain conditions. Some disorders and diseases can be traced to the inheritance of a single gene. Others depend on the inheritance of a group of genes or defective chromosomes. Knowledge about the genes that cause disease has led to research on gene therapy, which aims to give copies of the normal gene to the affected person.

Nurses need to understand the significance of inherited disease since many genetic diseases can be detected by genetic screening techniques in early embryos. Genetic screening is also assuming a greater importance in the assessment of risk for developing a disease in later life, e.g. some types of cancer and Alzheimer's disease.

Identification of the genes involved in disease will undoubtedly influence the way in which patients are treated in the future. Instead of treating and managing the nursing care of patients with end stage disease, people will be advised about treatments which could prevent the disease that they are most likely to inherit.

Genes

All the genetic information about an organism is passed from cell to cell via DNA in the nucleus. The DNA is arranged in genes on chromosomes. A chromosome is a linear DNA molecule bound with proteins called histones, which keep the chromosome tightly folded so that it fits into the nucleus.

Chromosomes

In humans there are 23 pairs of chromosomes. The sex chromosomes (X and Y) have different structures but each of the other pairs (autosomes) have similar structures. Normal female chromosomes are XX and normal male chromosomes are XY. It is possible to identify and count the number of chromosomes in a cell by special staining techniques. The results from these techniques are called the karyotype (Fig. 6.1).

Normal female

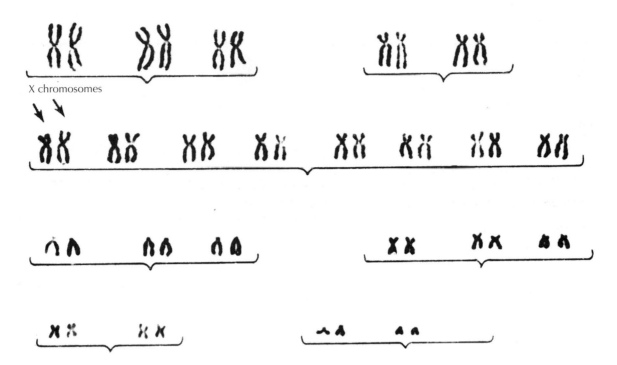

Fig. 6.1 Human chromosomes.

Remember that egg (ovum) and sperm cells only have one set of chromosomes as a result of meiosis. Therefore at fertilisation one set of chromosomes comes from the father and the other set from the mother. This allows different combinations of genes; a process called genetic recombination, so characteristics (traits) not found in either parent can be expressed in their children.

Identification of single genes

The human genome has about 30 000 genes arranged linearly on the chromosomes. Each gene has a particular place or locus on a chromosome and it is possible to identify them using special DNA fluorescent techniques, e.g. fluorescence in-situ hybridisation (FISH) uses a DNA sequence that will bind to a specific gene and also has a fluorescent dye attached to it.

When the DNA recognises the correct sequence on a chromosome the gene will be 'tagged' and can be identified by fluorescence microscopy.

Alleles

Although each gene codes for a specific characteristic (trait) not all genes are the same. This is because genes are made from two alleles, which code for the same characteristic, one from each parent. The alleles can be identical (homozygous) meaning that the alleles from each parent are the same or different (heterozygous) where the alleles from each parent are different. In Fig. 6.2 each gene codes for a trait that is only expressed if the gene is homozygous. Therefore, the person with these genes would be able to curl their tongue and wiggle their ears but not have dimples, illustrating how genetic variation in a population occurs.

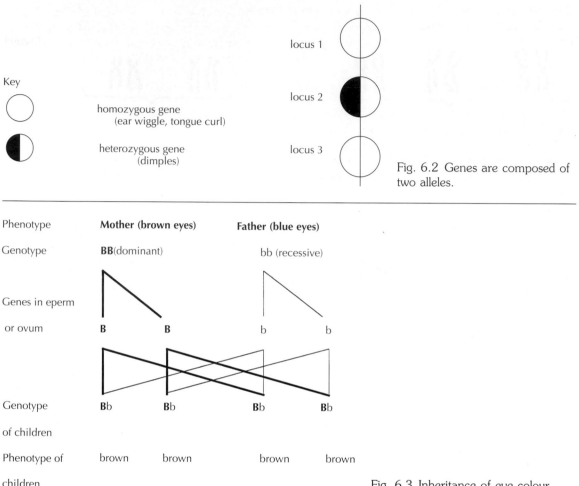

Key

○   homozygous gene
        (ear wiggle, tongue curl)

◐   heterozygous gene
        (dimples)

locus 1

locus 2

locus 3

Fig. 6.2 Genes are composed of two alleles.

Phenotype	**Mother (brown eyes)**	**Father (blue eyes)**		
Genotype	**BB**(dominant)	bb (recessive)		
Genes in eperm or ovum	**B** **B**	b b		
Genotype of children	**B**b **B**b	**B**b **B**b		
Phenotype of children	brown brown	brown brown		

Fig. 6.3 Inheritance of eye colour.

Dominant and recessive alleles

If one allele hides the expression of another at a single locus it is said to be dominant over the other recessive allele. An example is eye colour. The allele for brown eyes is dominant over the allele for blue eyes. This pattern of inheritance can be shown diagramatically (Fig. 6.3) where the mother and the father are both homozygous (two identical alleles) for eye colour but the father has blue eyes (b) and the mother brown eyes (B). Working through the diagram you should be able to see that the children can only be heterozygous (Bb) with brown eyes.

The dominant allele for brown colour (B) hides the effect of the recessive allele (b) for blue eye colour giving the phenotype (observable trait) brown eyes. However all of the chil-

Exercise 6.1

What do you think will be the eye colour (phenotype) of children born to a mother with Bb heterozygous genotype and a bb homozygous genotype father?

dren will carry a gene for blue eye colour and therefore have a heterozygous genotype for eye colour.

Polygenic inheritance

The fact that some of us have green eyes or different shades of brown or blue might make you doubt the simple illustration of dominant and recessive alleles above. This can be explained by the fact that many human traits are polygenic, meaning that more than one gene is involved in a single observable trait.

Eye colour actually involves many genes, which together synthesise melanin, a pigment that gives our eyes and skin their colour. Green and blue eyes have very little melanin whereas black and brown eyes have a lot. Height and intelligence are other examples of polygenic inheritance.

Co-dominance

Sometimes the polypeptide product from each allele interacts to produce different phenotypes. This relationship is described as co-dominance where the products of both alleles appear in the heterozygote. An example of co-dominance is shown in the four possible blood groups in humans (A, AB, B, O) which are determined by three alleles at a single locus I (I stands for isoagglutinogen, another name for antigen). I^A and I^B are co-dominant and both are dominant to I^l. Those who have A or B blood are heterozygous with I^l the third allele which is recessive and does not code for an antigen. People with O blood have two recessive alleles. People who have AB blood group have one allele coding for A antigen and one allele coding for B antigen on the red blood cell membrane, both of which are expressed (Table 6.1).

Gene inheritance patterns

It is possible to predict the chance of inheriting a gene by looking at pedigree charts that show genetic connections through generations. Pedigree charts help to identify whether a gene is carried on a sex chromosome (X or Y) or an autosome (a non-sex chromosome). They can also show whether a gene is dominant or recessive and if a person will be a carrier of a recessive gene that can be passed on to future generations. One of the most famous pedigree charts is that of the European royal families originating from Queen Victoria who was a carrier of haemophilia. One of her sons Leopold had haemophilia and died at the comparatively young age of 32. Two of her daughters, Alice of Hesse and Beatrice were carriers. The gene does not affect the present royal family because they are descendants of Edward VII, an unaffected child.

Pedigree charts

Pedigree charts or family trees are simply diagrams of a family structure. They are drawn up when an individual requests more information. This person is called the propositus or proposita depending on whether they are male or female respectively, they are indicated by an arrow in the chart. There are specific rules and symbols for drawing up a chart because they can become quite complex and interpretation would be more difficult if the same symbols were not applied (Fig. 6.4).

Generations are written on the same line with the first born starting from the left. A Roman numeral or a letter indicates each generation so individuals can be referred to as A.2 or I.2. A pedigree chart for an autosomal recessive disease is shown in Fig. 6.5.

Table 6.1 Human blood groups

Genotype	Phenotype (blood group)
I^A I^B	AB
I^A I^A or I^A I^l	A
I^B I^B or I^B I^l	B
I^l I^l	O

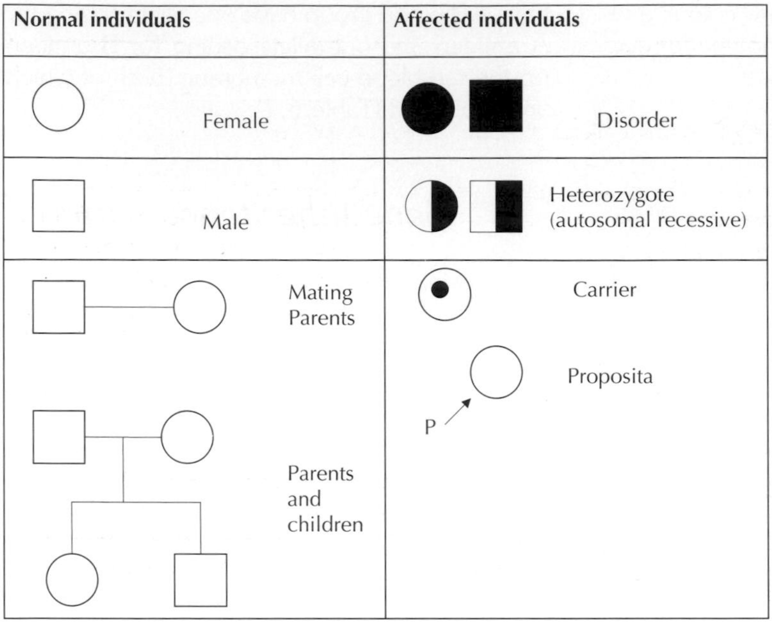

Normal individuals		Affected individuals	
○	Female	● ■	Disorder
□	Male	◐ ◧	Heterozygote (autosomal recessive)
□—○	Mating Parents	◉	Carrier
□—○ with children	Parents and children	P ↗ ○	Proposita

Fig. 6.4 Symbols for pedigree charts.

Activity

Draw up your family tree using the appropriate symbols.

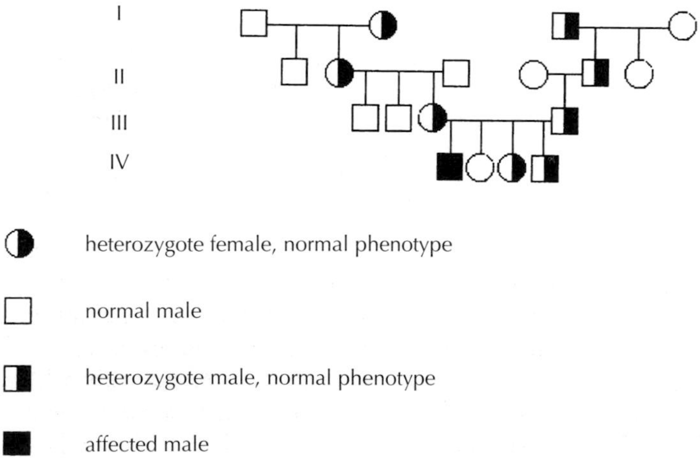

◐ heterozygote female, normal phenotype

□ normal male

◧ heterozygote male, normal phenotype

■ affected male

Fig. 6.5 Pedigree chart for an autosomal recessive disease.

A nurse could be asked to help a patient gather information for a pedigree chart or explain their use to affected individuals. The charts give a picture of the spread of a genetic trait throughout a family that can be more easily understood. However it is important to realise that the trait may not always be expressed in the same way in an individual family member.

Table 6.2 Genetic disorders

Genetic disorder	Definition	Example
Single gene	One or more mutant alleles at each locus	Cystic fibrosis
Multifactorial inheritance	Trait caused by both genes and environmental factors	Congenital malformations, e.g. congenital heart disease, cleft lip and palate; common disorders of adult life, e.g. schizophrenia, diabetes mellitus
Chromosomal disorders	Changes to the number or structure of the cell chromosomes	Down's syndrome, fragile X syndrome

Genetic disorders

Genetic disorders are the result of changes in DNA mutation which can be inherited because the mutation is present in either the ovum or sperm cells. They can conveniently be placed in three categories, single gene disorders caused by a change in the DNA for an allele, multifactorial disorders caused by changes to the genes and environmental factors and chromosomal abnormalities which involve either the number or structure of chromosomes (Table 6.2). As our knowledge about genetics increases there is no doubt that these broad groups will be further refined.

Single gene disorders

Genetic disorders, which can easily be traced through generations, are normally single gene disorders, i.e. only one gene is not working properly. This group of diseases follow specific patterns as originally predicted by Gregor Mendel, the first classical geneticist. His observations made it possible to calculate the risk of having the disorder in future generations and this is often referred to as Mendelian inheritance.

Multifactorial disorders

The more we understand about genetics and genetically related disorders, the more we have

Table 6.3 Heritability of single gene and multifactorial disorders

Single gene	Multifactorial
Risk is the same at birth as in later life	Risk increases throughout life
Phenotype is predictable	Phenotype is variable
Possession of the mutant genotype results in disease	Possession of a threshold level of mutant genes is needed for the disease to result

come to realise that in humans many diseases are caused by a combination of environmental factors and a number of genes. The risk of developing such multifactorial diseases is difficult to predict compared with single gene disorders.

The relative importance of the genetic contribution to such diseases rather than the environmental factors is called heritability, e.g. schizophrenia has a heritability of 85% which means that relatives of a person with schizophrenia have a high chance of developing it also. A low heritability indicates that relatives are less likely to be affected.

The differences between the heritability of single gene disorders and multifactorial disorders are shown in Table 6.3 and a list of multifactorial disorders and their heritability in Table

Table 6.4 Multifactorial diseases and their heritability

Disease	Heritability (%)
Asthma	80
Schizophrenia	85
Arteriosclerosis	65
Hypertension (essential)	62
Congenital dislocation of the hip	60
Alzheimer's disease (AD2 late onset)	40–50
Peptic ulcer	37

6.4. The wide range of heritability, schizophrenia 85% to peptic ulcer 37%, shows that environmental factors play a greater part in the development of peptic ulcers than in schizoprenia.

Many of these figures have been derived from studies with twins, particularly identical twins, who have been brought up separately. In this case the environmental and genetic contribution can be clearly defined. A study of identical twins showed that the incidence of insulin-dependent diabetes was 50% but in non-insulin-dependent diabetes mellitus the incidence was 90%. This indicates that genetic factors were significant in both forms of diabetes but that environmental factors were more important in the development of insulin-dependent diabetes.

The influence of the environment on the expression of our genes forms the basis of the 'nature' and 'nurture' debate. Are we fat because of our genes or simply because we eat too much? What is the relationship of our genes with alcoholism, sexual orientation or diet? Conjecture is endless because scientific evidence is difficult to obtain and as yet tends to raise more questions rather than providing an answer.

As you would expect, multifactorial diseases are much more difficult to predict in future generations. Preparing pedigree charts is of limited use but study of these charts has shown that a disease can be dependent on whether the gene

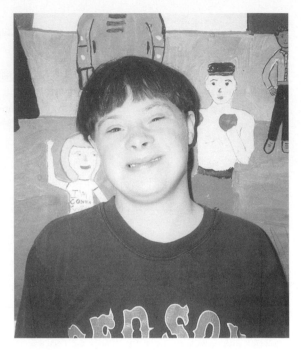

Fig. 6.6 Typical facial characteristics of Down's syndrome.

has been inherited from the mother or father. This is called genomic imprinting. Interestingly, it would seem that some childhood cancers can be explained in this way.

Chromosomal abnormalities

Chromosome abnormalities cause many genetic diseases and include changes both in the number of chromosomes and to the structure of the chromosome itself. Chromosomal abnormalities occur in about 7.5% of conceptions but about 0.5–1% of live births. About half of spontaneous miscarriages can be attributed to chromosomal abnormality.

Changes in chromosome number are caused by the chromosomes not separating properly at meiosis or mitosis, e.g. Down's syndrome (Fig. 6.6), is due to three 21 chromosomes (trisomy 21) which seem to be strongly linked to the age of the mother but the link with age is not common to all chromosome disorders.

Table 6.5 Chromosomal abnormalities

Disease	Cause	Incidence
Down's syndrome	Trisomy 21	1 in 650 births, incidence increases with maternal age
Fragile X syndrome	Codon repeat on X chromosome	1 in 2000 males
Huntington's chorea	Codon repeat on chromosome 4	1 in 10 000
Turner's syndrome	No Y chromosome	1 in 2500 females

Fragile X syndrome is a result of too many copies of a codon (trinucleotide repeats) on the X chromosome. It is the most common cause of mental retardation that is inherited. The pattern of inheritance is different from X-linked inheritance in that the grandsons of some apparently unaffected males are affected so the generation is important here. Examples of chromosomal abnormalities are shown in Table 6.5. It is interesting that some of them, e.g. Huntingdon's chorea, are also autosomal dominant disorders.

Characteristics of single-gene disorders

There are over 6000 single-gene traits and disorders affecting between 1 and 2% of the population. The inheritance patterns of these disorders are well established and have shown that different populations have a different incidence of this type of disease. For example, in the Caucasian population of the UK, cystic fibrosis is relatively common whereas β thalassaemia occurs more frequently in Mediterranean and SE Asian populations. This means that these populations can be targeted for genetic testing.

Autosomal recessive inheritance

Autosomal recessive inheritance is only seen when the defective or mutant allele is present in both parents. The parents can be perfectly healthy but carry the mutant gene or could

suffer from the disease itself. Generally the parents do not have a homozygous genotype. Tracing a disorder through the family is usually not possible because all the affected individuals are in a single generation, i.e. brothers and sisters.

In very rare disorders, parents are often related and consequently will have many genes in common. Studies of the parents of children with alcaptonuria, a metabolic disorder in which homogentisic acid is excreted in the urine, which goes dark on exposure to air, and a dark pigment is deposited in the cartilage and joints, showed that more than a quarter of them were first cousins (consanguinity). When the disease is more common as in cystic fibrosis, there is a greater incidence of the gene in the general population and the significance of parents being first cousins is minimal.

Cystic fibrosis

Cystic fibrosis is a multisystem disease characterised by the production of sticky mucus in the lungs and pancreas. Improved management of the disease has increased life expectancy to about 50 years. Chest physiotherapy to remove sticky mucus from the lungs is an essential part of the treatment. These children are prone to infections, particularly chronic bacterial infections (e.g. *Pseudomonas aeruginosa* infections).

Children born with the disease have parents who are both heterozygous for the gene. The probability of having an affected child is 1 in 4, a carrier child 1 in 2 and a non-affected child

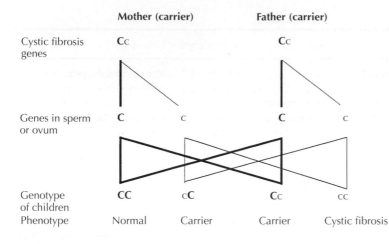

Fig. 6.7 Pattern of inheritance for cystic fibrosis (autosomal recessive inheritance).

Table 6.6 Autosomal recessive disorders

Disorder	Symptoms	Detection
Phenylketonuria (PKU)	Decreased IQ, fits, eczema	Guthrie heel prick test in newborn
Sickle cell disease	Homozygotes: sickle cell anaemia, sickle cell crises.	Pre-natal diagnosis
	Heterozygotes: sickle cell trait, resistance to malaria	
Tay-Sachs disease	Progressive neurological abnormalities. Death 3–5 years of age	Carrier screening, prenatal diagnosis
α and β thalassaemia	Haemolytic anaemia and compensatory hyperplasia of the bone marrow	Haemoglobin analysis. Ultrasound fetus scan for severe α thalassaemia

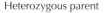

Fig. 6.8 A Punnett's square.

1 in 4, (Fig. 6.7). In the UK the probability of being a carrier is $1:25$ and the incidence 1 in 2500 live births.

A Punnett's square (Fig. 6.8) could be constructed to show the same information, i.e. heterozygous parents could produce children with a 1 in 4 chance of having the disease. It is important to remember when making this kind of risk assessment that the chance or probability of having an affected child is the same for each pregnancy. Having one affected child does not improve the chance of having an unaffected child.

The Punnett's square illustrates the possible recombinations that can occur in a simple format. Heterozygous parents for cystic fibrosis have a 1 in 4 chance of having an affected child (**cc**).

Other autosomal recessive diseases with the same pattern of inheritance are listed in Table 6.6.

Sickle cell trait is also an example of co-dominance. Mutant haemoglobin (Hb), which

Table 6.7 X-linked recessive disorders

Disorder	Incidence	Symptoms	Detection
Haemophilia A	1 in 10 000 males	Haemorrhage into joints and soft tissues; decreased life expectancy	Prenatal fetal sampling; DNA analysis, pedigree chart
Haemophilia B (Christmas disease)	1 in 30 000 males	Haemorrhage as in A but less severe; decreased life expectancy	Prenatal fetal sampling; DNA analysis, pedigree chart
Duchenne muscular dystrophy	1 in 3500 males	30% decreased IQ, symmetrical wasting of muscle tissue; death at around 20 years due to respiratory failure	DNA analysis, blood creatine kinase values very high
Becker muscular dystrophy	1 in 30 000 males	Wheelchair bound at 16 years; near normal life expectancy	DNA analysis, blood creatine kinase raised

causes the red blood cells to change shape 'sickle' at low oxygen concentrations and normal haemoglobin are both synthesised in heterozygotes because the gene has one normal and one mutant allele.

X-linked recessive inheritance

Sex linked gene disorders are primarily carried by the X chromosome but rare examples of Y-linked inheritance do exist. Remember that a male has one X and one Y chromosome and a female two X chromosomes. The male with a defective or mutant allele on his X chromosome is homozygous for that allele. Examples of these disorders are shown in Table 6.7. One of the best known examples of this type of disease is haemophilia.

Haemophilia

There are two kinds of haemophilia both of which are X-linked. Haemophilia A is the most common (Table 6.7). The defective gene codes for clotting factor VIII but in haemophilia B the defective clotting factor is factor IX, this is often called Christmas disease. Only males are affected and they can die from untreated bruises

		Xh	X	Carrier female (**XhX**)
Normal male	X	**XhX**	XX	
	Y	**XhY**	XY	

Fig. 6.9 Haemophilia X-linked inheritance from carrier females and normal males.

or internal bleeding; however, females are carriers of the disease.

Inheritance pattern

Haemophilia and all X-linked recessive gene diseases are characterised by the fact that more males than females are affected. Carrier females who appear healthy keep the disease in the population. Their children have a 50% chance of being carriers if female and the same chance of having the disorder if male (Fig. 6.9). However in about one-third of families there is no history of haemophilia and it is assumed that these are caused by spontaneous mutation of the gene.

Haemophiliac males do not pass the disease to their sons, but all their daughters will be carriers (Fig. 6.10).

Normal female \ Haemophiliac male	**Xh**	Y
X	X**Xh**	XY
X	X**Xh**	XY

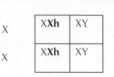

Fig. 6.10 Inheritance pattern for haemophiliac male with unaffected female.

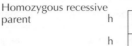

Homozygous recessive parent \ Heterozygous parent	**H**	h
h	**H**h	hh
h	**H**h	hh

Huntington's chorea

Fig. 6.11 Pattern of inheritance for autosomal dominant genes.

Activity

Find a family tree for Queen Victoria and confirm that the facts are true for this case.

Autosomal dominant inheritance

How can we tell if a disease is the result of inheritance of a dominant gene? The first clue is that it will be present in every generation because even if the genotype is heterozygous the dominant gene will be expressed. Therefore there is a 1 : 2 chance that the child of heterozygous and homozygous recessive parents will have an affected child (Fig. 6.11).

Huntington's chorea

You might think that autosomal dominant diseases can only be very mild because the genes have survived in the population but this is not the case. The gene pool is sustained because many of the diseases do not appear until later in life after the affected person has had children. Huntington's chorea is an example. About 7 people per 100 000 in the UK suffer in all racial groups. It is interesting that the disease which appears before the age of 20 is nearly always passed on from the father, but later onset (around 40) is passed on by the mother – another example of genomic imprinting. Homozygous embryos die, only heterozygotes survive.

The defective gene leads to the degeneration of the brain basal cell nuclei causing convulsive movement and loss of brain function followed by death. The aim of health care for the patients is relief of symptoms initially by drugs but later to ensure that the patient retains their dignity until death. Living with the knowledge that you will develop the disease presents many problems. Nursing present and possible future patients requires a clear supportive and sensitive approach.

Penetrance

More examples of autosomal dominant diseases are shown in Table 6.8. Polydactyly is an example of incomplete penetrance. Penetrance is a term used to explain why a faulty gene is expressed in some individuals and not others. For example 100% penetration is shown by cystic fibrosis but polydactyly is incompletely penetrant, some babies who have the gene will have the correct number of fingers and others additional ones. Often parents are surprised when their baby has additional fingers and have no memory of the condition in their families. This is because the extra digits are usually removed very soon after birth.

Three clinical subtypes of Alzheimer's disease are autosomal dominant mutations but account for less than 1% of cases.

Table 6.8 Examples of autosomal dominant diseases

Disease	Incidence	Symptoms	Detection
Huntington's chorea	1 in 10 000	Personality changes, dementia; progressive chorea	Genetic testing, magnetic resonance imaging (MRI)
Familial hypercholesterolaemia	1 in 500	At 30–40 years, ischaemic heart disease; homozygous children can die in early adulthood	Very high blood cholesterol; DNA analysis
Achondroplasia	1 in 10 000	Dwarfism; normal IQ, normal life expectancy	Fetal ultrasound
Polydactyly	Not determined	Extra fingers or toes	Fetal ultrasound
Retinoblastoma	1 in 18 000	Tumour of the eye, onset in first two years	Squint

Table 6.9 Autosomal dominant pattern of inheritance for some common cancers

Disorder	Cancer	Gene
Familial breast/ovarian cancer	Breast, ovary	BRCA1
Familial breast cancer	Breast	BRCA2
Hereditary non-polyposis colon cancer	Colon, endometrium	MSH2, MLH1, PMS1
Familial adenomatous polyposis	Colorectal	APC
Retinoblastoma	Eye, bone	Rb

Cancer

There is a huge public interest in the possible genetic links for cancer. This is partly because it has been shown that some common cancers e.g. breast, ovarian and colorectal cancer show an autosomal dominant pattern of inheritance (Table 6.9).

Genes that cause cancer are called oncogenes. These do not normally cause tumour formation because other genes, for example suppressor genes, prevent them from being expressed. However if either the oncogenes or suppressor genes become damaged in any way, cell division is no longer controlled and cancer results. It looks as though all autosomal domi-

Table 6.10 Difference between oncogenes and tumour suppressor genes

Tumour suppressor gene	Oncogene
Mutations can be inherited	Mutations rarely inherited
Inactive in tumour	Active in tumour
Associated with leukaemia and lymphomas	Associated with solid tumours

nant hereditary cancers are due to mutated tumour suppressor genes. The differences between these and oncogenes are shown in Table 6.10.

A tumour suppressive gene called *p53* on chromosome 17 seems to be important in a wide range of cancers. A mutated form of the gene seems to activate the development of cancer. Screening for this gene can therefore be used as a diagnostic tool and more excitingly is a potential candidate for gene therapy.

Nevertheless, the vast majority of cancers do not show this particular pattern of inheritance. Environmental factors (e.g. radiation or chemical) causing the DNA to mutate are far more significant. At the same time, understanding the function of the genes involved in cell division and its control can only help towards providing a means of prevention or cure.

Genetic techniques

Gene therapy

Gene therapy is the transfer of normal copies of a gene into an individual, in the hope that the individual will then be able to synthesise copies of the normal protein. This fairly simple concept depends on making sufficient copies of the gene, which can be targeted to the right tissue and does not get into egg or sperm cells (germ-line cells) so that the 'foreign' gene cannot be passed on to future generations – a 'tall order'!

Gene therapy has had some success with the treatment of cystic fibrosis. The gene for cystic fibrosis has been identified. Normal copies of the gene have been put (cloned) into a vector (carrier) so that it can be transported into the patient. The vector has to be very small and is usually a virus, which will enter specific cells. In the case of cystic fibrosis an inactivated adenovirus has been used as a vector because it infects the human respiratory tract. The patient inhales the vector suspension and the virus enters the epithelial cells and expresses the normal gene. Unfortunately, the cells die after a few months as dictated by their normal cell cycle so the capacity to synthesise a normal copy of the defective gene is lost, making further treatments necessary.

Another example is using normal copies of the human suppressor *p53* gene as a complementary therapy to chemotherapy and radiotherapy for cancer because it is the most commonly mutated gene in many cancers.

Gene therapy might seem to be the perfect treatment if not a cure for inherited diseases. Identification and cloning of the genes is becoming easier to achieve but finding an appropriate vector is more problematic. Nevertheless it is likely that more diseases will be treated in this way in the future.

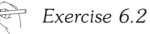

Exercise 6.2

The *nm* 23 gene is believed to act as a metastasis suppressor gene (stops cancer cells from spreading) in breast cancer. If this gene is not expressed a poor survival rate is indicated. How could this information be used for potential treatment of breast cancer?

Prenatal genetic testing

Demand for prenatal testing has grown as the safety of the techniques and their reliability have improved. The techniques available vary from completely non-invasive ultrasound to taking samples of fetal blood, which represents a greater risk. Prenatal genetic testing methods are summarised in Table 6.11.

Amniocentesis

This technique samples the amniotic fluid surrounding the fetus using an aspiration

Table 6.11 Prenatal genetic testing methods

Technique	Week of pregnancy	Use	Risk to fetus
Ultrasound	16–18 weeks	Monitoring of fetal growth, development of abnormalities, e.g. polydactyly, heart defects	None
Amniocentesis	16–18 weeks	Karyotyping, fetal sex; fluid analysis for enzymes and AFP[+]	Low: 1% above normal
Chorionic villus sampling	8–10 weeks	DNA analysis and cell karyotype	2–3% above the average
Fetal blood sampling (cardiocentesis)	18 weeks and later	Single-gene disorders, fragile X, suspected fetal infection	1–2%, rhesus (Rh) immunisation if mother is Rh negative
Maternal blood sampling	16–18 weeks	TORCH[*] screen for infections that cause congenital malformations. Triple test[++] for risk of neural tube defects (e.g. spina bifida) and Down's syndrome	0%
Pre implantation diagnosis for in-vitro fertilisation (IVF)	0 weeks	Detecting X-linked disorders or known at-risk genetic disorder.	0%

[+]alpha feto-protein.
[*]TORCH: toxoplasmosis, other agents, rubella, cytomegalovirus, herpes simplex.
[++]Triple test: serum AFP, human chorionic gonadotrophin (HCG), oestradiol.

needle (Fig. 6.12). The fluid can be analysed for enzymes and alpha feto-protein (AFP) which helps to detect neural tube defects such as spina bifida. The fetal cells in the fluid can be analysed for specific DNA sequences or grown in culture for chromosome analysis (karyotyping).

Of the invasive techniques, amniocentesis is the safest and most medical experience is with this technique. Both amniotic fluid and fetal cells are available for analysis. The disadvantage of the method is that it is performed at 16–20 weeks, which leaves little time for repeat tests and parental decision.

Chorionic villus sampling

Chorionic villus sampling takes a small sample of placental tissue, which contains fetal cells. Sampling is carried out earlier in pregnancy at 8–12 weeks and gives time for amniocentesis later if the results are inconclusive. The disadvantage is that no fluid is obtained for AFP analysis and limb abnormalities may occur in the baby.

Table 7.1 Common microorganisms

Name	Type
Escherichia coli	Bacterium
Staphylococcus aureus	Bacterium
Pseudomonas aeruginosa	Bacterium
Streptococcus pneumoniae	Bacterium
Clostridium perfringens	Bacterium
Mycobacterium tuberculosis	Bacterium
Candida albicans	Yeast
Mucor spp.	Mould
Aspergillus fumigatus	Mould
Influenza	Virus
Herpes	Virus

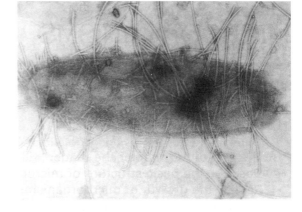

Fig. 7.2 Electron micrograph of a Gram-negative bacterium with flagella and fimbriae.

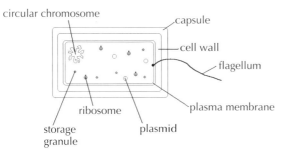

Fig. 7.1 Structure of a bacterial cell.

layer is present or not. The function of the cell wall is to maintain the relatively high pressure in the cell caused by the concentration of dissolved solutes and also to give the cell shape and rigidity.

Capsules and slime layers

Outside the cell wall some bacteria have either a capsule or a slime layer, which is sometimes called the glycocalyx. These sticky layers have an important role in attachment to cells and surfaces. They also help bacterial cells to stick to each other. Cells that are capsulated are frequently resistant to phagocytosis because the

white blood cells can not stick to the bacterium allowing the bacteria to grow and establish an infection, e.g. *Streptococcus pneumoniae*, which causes pneumonia.

Flagella, fimbriae and pili

Motile bacteria have a single flagellum or many flagella depending on the species. Motility helps the bacteria to move in a liquid towards food or away from harmful chemicals by a process called chemotaxis. Fimbriae are structurally similar to flagella but are shorter. They help bacteria to stick to specific human tissues or to each other (Fig. 7.2). Pili have a role in the bacterial reproduction process and act as a receptor for viruses.

Cytoplasmic structures

The cytoplasm is surrounded by a plasma membrane and contains all the structures necessary for life. Some bacteria have distinct internal membranes but these do not surround organelles.

DNA

The arrangement of DNA in bacteria is quite different from that in human cells. The bacterial chromosome is a single, closed, circular DNA molecule, which is folded and twisted (super coiled) to fit in the cell cytoplasm. It varies in size according to the type of bacterium, e.g. *Escherichia coli* has 5–8 times more DNA than *Chlamydia* spp. Some bacteria contain extra circles of DNA called plasmids. Plasmids replicate independently of the nuclear DNA and can be transferred from one bacterium to another. Sometimes they insert themselves into the bacterial chromosome and become part of the inherited information of the bacterium.

Ribosomes and storage granules

Bacterial ribosomes are smaller than those in human cells but have the same function in protein synthesis. Like human ribosomes they are composed of large and small subunits but they are not associated with membranes and are found in the cytoplasm. Storage granules are also found in the cytoplasm. The most common storage granules are polyhydroxybutyrate (PHB) and glycogen, which act as an energy and a carbon store.

Moulds and yeasts

Moulds and yeast are fungi. The basic structural unit of a mould is a thread like hypha which absorbs nutrients (Fig. 7.3a). Most hyphae are divided by cross walls which can be perforated by a central pore large enough to allow nuclei and organelles to move freely. The hyphae often fuse together to form a mycelium. Each hypha has a strong cell wall, which grows from the tip. Moulds produce thousands of spores from aerial hyphae (Fig. 7.3b) but yeasts reproduce by division or budding (Fig. 7.3c). Sometimes the buds do not separate from the mother cell and form a filament, e.g. *Candida albicans*.

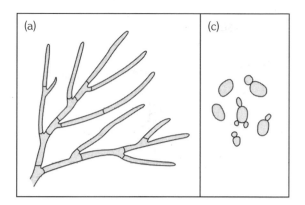

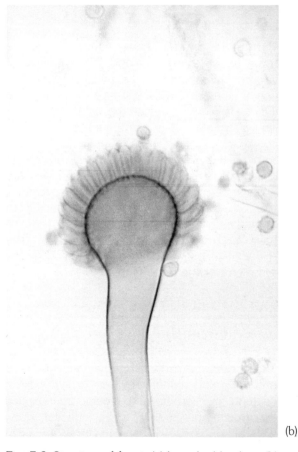

Fig. 7.3 Structure of fungi. (a) branched hyphae, (b) aerial hypha of *Aspergillus fumigatus*, (c) budding yeasts.

Viruses

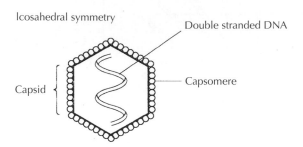

Fig. 7.4 Basic structure of a virus.

Viruses are smaller than bacteria. There are three basic structural shapes or symmetry of viruses, helical, polyhedral and complex. The genetic material is a single type of nucleic acid (DNA or RNA) that can be either double or single stranded. It is surrounded by a protein coat (capsid) made up of subunits called capsomeres (Fig. 7.4). The nucleic acid and protein coat, which make up the virus are called the nucleocapsid. Some viruses, e.g. influenza virus, have an outer membranous envelope, which originates from the host cell, but the proteins have been replaced by virus proteins. The structure of these viruses is determined by the symmetry of the nucleocapsid.

Growth

Microorganisms grow when they have the right nutrients and conditions for growth. Most bacteria are aerobic and require free oxygen for growth, but anaerobic bacteria can grow without oxygen. These can grow in deep wounds where the tissues are dead, e.g. *Clostridium tetani*. Facultatively anaerobic bacteria can grow with or without oxygen, e.g. *Escherichia coli* and *Pseudomonas aeruginosa*. Yeasts and moulds are generally aerobic and usually grow at lower temperatures and pH than bacteria.

Measuring growth

Microorganisms grow quickly compared with animals and plants. Their small size means that measuring their growth by an increase in size and weight is difficult. Therefore growth is measured in terms of the number of cells or the number of virus particles in a population.

Bacteria

Most bacteria grow by a process called binary fission. This means that the cell splits into two identical cells which in turn grow and divide to produce four cells, then eight, sixteen, thirty-two and so on (Fig. 7.5). This process can take as little as 20 minutes, e.g. *Escherichia coli* or many hours, e.g. *Mycobacterium* spp. but always results in large numbers (hundreds of millions per ml fluid). The difference in growth rates is reflected in the incubation period for a disease, i.e. the time taken for the bacterium to reach sufficient numbers from infection to cause symptoms of a disease.

When the nutrients run out or the conditions change, bacteria will stop growing. Some bacteria can form endospores, highly resistant structures, in these conditions. They can survive for years and are very difficult to kill, e.g. *Clostridium* spp. (Fig. 7.6).

Exercise 7.1

How many bacteria will there be after 1 hour starting with two bacteria which double every 15 minutes? Drawing the cells will make it easier.

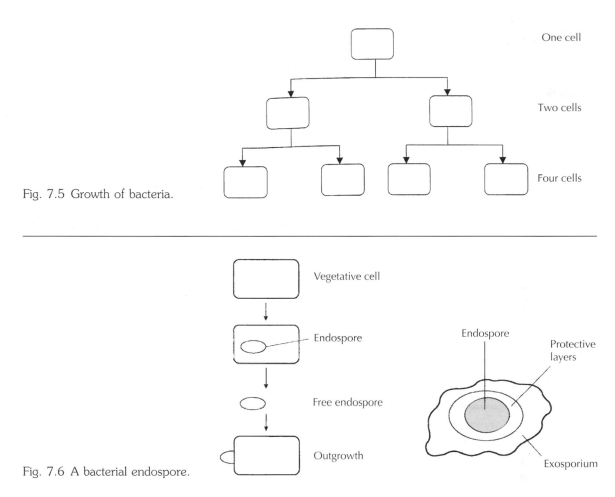

Fig. 7.5 Growth of bacteria.

Fig. 7.6 A bacterial endospore.

Yeasts and moulds

Most yeasts grow by a budding process whereby new cells form as a small outgrowth or bud of the mother cell. The bud enlarges and then separates. *Candida albicans* is a yeast which can also grow as a filament (Fig. 7.7). This type of growth is important for pathogenicity.

Moulds, *e.g. Aspergillus* and *Mucor* spp. grow by absorbing nutrients through their hyphae to produce a mat-like mycelium which spreads over the surface and then produces aerial spore-bearing structures. The spores are often coloured which gives the colonies their characteristic colour, *e.g.* moulds on bread are often a bluish green colour. Each microscopic spore is capable of growing into a new colony (Fig. 7.3b).

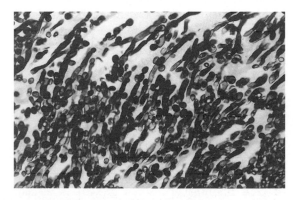

Fig. 7.7 *Candida albicans* in the tissue of a heart valve.

Viruses

Viruses grow by attacking and entering a host cell, if the cell is a bacterium the virus is called a bacteriophage. The virus makes the cell synthesise viral proteins and nucleic acid, which are then assembled into new virus particles. The release of the viruses usually causes cell destruction, e.g. influenza virus but some viruses, e.g. herpes, just weaken the host cell because they are only released from the host cell intermittently by budding out of the cell membrane.

Laboratory techniques

Bacteria are grown in the laboratory from the swabs taken from patients. The swabs will usually contain a mixture of bacteria so first of all they have to be separated to obtain a pure culture. This is not as difficult as it might seem because each bacterium will grow on different nutrients or tolerate different conditions, which will separate them into different groups.

Culturing microorganisms

Bacteria are grown on a jelly-like substance called agar in a petri dish. The swab is spread over the surface of the agar (plated out) and incubated at 37 °C for about 24 h. A single dot of bacteria or colony containing thousands of the same bacteria are then removed and used to inoculate a liquid nutrient medium to grow. Growth is detected as a cloudy suspension. This process takes quite a long time and is the reason why results from laboratory tests can take 48 h and sometimes longer. Fungi are cultured in the same way but grow more slowly and require different nutrients, lower temperatures and pH than bacteria.

Human viruses can be grown on a single layer of cells (monolayer). Virus growth is usually detected because it destroys or inhibits the growth of the cell, which can be seen as a clear area called a plaque. Each plaque is considered to originate from one virus particle. Sometimes the cells are not destroyed, e.g. tumour viruses make the cells grow more quickly and pile up to form a focus of growth or infection. Alternatively, virus growth can be measured by counting the number of antibodies produced by the host in response to an infection.

Laboratory tests to identify microorganisms

The name of a bacterium tells you something about it. For example, the genus name *Staphylococcus* tells us that the bacterium is a Gram-positive coccus which groups together in grape-like clusters, the species (denoted by sp. (singular) or spp. (plural)) name *aureus* tells us that the colonies are a golden colour. However there are different strains of the same species. Therefore there are many different *Escherichia coli*, not all of them are pathogenic (capable of causing disease) but some can cause fatal food poisoning. Similarly *Staphylococcus aureus* can be a harmless commensal bacterium on your skin but if it is resistant to antibiotics and is transferred to a patient it could cause a fatal infection.

Different strains would be impossible to distinguish from each other simply by looking at them under a microscope. They have to be cultured or grown in large numbers so that tests can be carried out to identify them. Identification of strains is really important when trying to trace the origin of an outbreak of an epidemic. Common laboratory tests include counting the total number of bacteria in 1 mL of fluid sample and staining to show evidence of infection either from pure cultures or from pieces of tissues.

Gram stain

One of the most common stains used to help to identify bacteria is the Gram stain. It divides bacteria into two groups, depending on the cell wall reaction to the dyes safranin or crystal

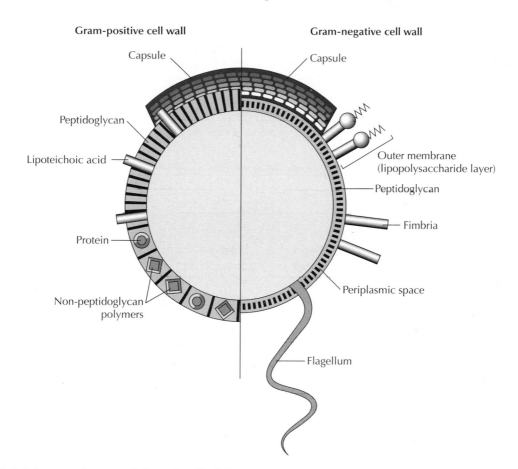

Fig. 7.8 Schematic diagram of the cell wall of Gram-negative and Gram-positive bacteria.

violet. Bacteria staining purple from the crystal violet are Gram-positive, e.g. *Clostridium perfringens*, *Staphylococcus aureus* whereas those which lose the stain when washed with alcohol but retain the pink safranin stain are called Gram-negative, e.g. *Escherichia coli*, *Pseudomonas aeruginosa* (Fig. 7.8). Some bacteria do not Gram stain, e.g. *Mycobacterium* spp., because their cell walls contain a lot of lipids, an acid-fast stain is used to identify them. The bacterial cells stain pink but tissue cells stain green.

Staining bacteria makes it possible to look at their shape under the light microscope. Shape can also be used to help identify bacteria (Fig. 7.9), e.g. spherical (cocci), rod-shaped (bacilli), comma-like (vibrio).

Yeasts and moulds cannot be Gram stained and are usually identified by staining the infected tissue and looking for typical structures. Pure cultures can be stained with cotton blue to reveal the reproductive structures.

Viruses are too small to be viewed directly under a light microscope therefore special immunogenic stains are used which 'label' the virus so their presence can be detected in cells; sometimes they are viewed directly under an electron microscope.

Infection

An infection occurs when microorganisms grow and overcome the resistance mechanisms of the

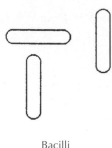

Bacilli

Cocco-bacilli

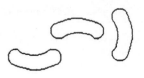

Comma shaped
bacilli

Fig. 7.9 Some shapes of bacterial cells.

body. If they harm or damage the body they are called pathogens. A pathogen must grow in the body to produce an infection. Virulence is a term used to describe the number of microorganisms needed to give rise to an infection. The microorganisms grow either throughout the body (systemic infections) or are restricted to an area, e.g. boils and abscesses. In systemic infections the microorganisms are spread via the blood. The terms used to describe bacterial infections are:

- bacteraemia: when bacteria growing in tissues are detected in the blood
- septicaemia: when bacteria grow and divide in the blood
- pyaemia: bacteria and white cells forming pus are detected in the blood.

Some infecting microorganisms produce toxins. Exotoxins are secreted from bacteria as they grow. They can travel and cause damage to the body at sites remote from the initial infection, e.g. tetanus toxin causes spastic paralysis but enters the body usually via a puncture wound. Endotoxins are part of the cell wall of Gram-negative bacteria and are only released when the cells die, e.g. Salmonella toxin.

Hospital acquired infections (HAIs)

It seems incredible that infections acquired during a hospital stay are more common than having a traffic accident and cost millions of pounds for additional treatment from longer stays in hospital. These infections can be called nosocomial infections (from the Latin word nosocomium for hospital). Aseptic technique describes the methods used to try and prevent patients acquiring hospital infections. The technique is used for any invasive procedure and equipment such as urinary catheters used for the procedures. Infection control teams put procedures in place to minimise the risk of infection but it is thought that about 30% of current HAIs are preventable. National guidelines for the prevention and control of HAIs were published in 2001. They include sets of recommendations for the following categories: standard principles for all healthcare practitioners, short-term indwelling urethral catheters and central venous catheters.

Routes of infection

How do patients become infected when they are in hospital? Infections result when microorganisms are spread from a reservoir of infection to the susceptible host. Routes of infection are shown in Table 7.2. The reservoir of infection, i.e. anywhere microorganisms can survive and multiply, can be either from the patients themselves (self-infection) or from other patients, visitors or hospital staff (cross-infection).

Table 7.2 Routes of infection

Route of spread (transmission)	Example
Contact	Contaminated hands, equipment, clothing
Aerosols	Inhalation of dust, skin scales in air, water droplets from humidifiers or nebulisers
Blood	Inoculation accidents, mother to baby (prenatal), sexual activity
Food/water	Ingestion of viruses and bacteria or toxins from them in food or water
Insects	Cockroaches carrying pathogens can contaminate sterile supplies or food

Self-infection occurs when tissues become infected from a different site in the patient's body, e.g. upper respiratory tract, gastrointestinal (alimentary) tract and skin.

Cross infections can arise from people suffering from an infection or who are symptomless carriers or from a 'reservoir of infection'.

Prevention of infection

A key role of the nurse is to know the procedures and practices which are most likely to cause HALs, e.g. invasive techniques, line manipulations, and to realise that other factors such as poor cleaning, poor patient nutrition and immunosuppression can increase the risk of infection. Probably the most important preventative factor is ensuring that the time is taken to carry out the infection control procedures, which are in place in every hospital. Barrier nursing attempts to stop the spread of infections by protective isolation or to prevent the spread of infection from infected patients (source isolation).

Hygiene measures for procedures at risk of causing HAIs

Hand washing

Hand washing is a cheap and important routine infection control procedure and the best method to prevent the transmission of microorganisms. It has been shown that it significantly reduces infection rates in intensive care units and gastrointestinal infections. Damaged skin on the hands has a higher number of pathogens responsible for HAIs.

The key factors that promote good hygiene and maintain skin integrity are:

- the time taken to wash your hands
- exposure of all areas of the hands and wrists to the preparation being used
- vigorous rubbing to create friction
- thorough rinsing
- ensuring that the hands are completely dry.

Transient bacteria can be almost completely removed with soap and water but have little effect against resident bacteria. Bactericidal hand washes, e.g. Hibiscrub®, Povidone–iodine®, make the procedure more effective in removing resident bacteria. Attention to areas where microorganisms collect, e.g. between the fingers is important (Fig. 7.10).

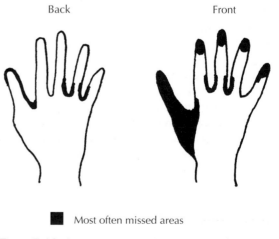

Back   Front

■ Most often missed areas

Fig. 7.10 Areas commonly missed following handwashing.

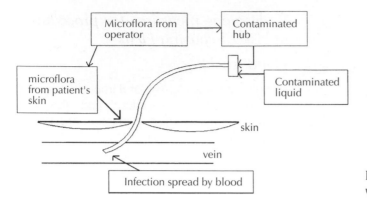

Fig. 7.11 Routes of infection associated with IV devices.

However, even using a bactericide, will not remove *all* bacteria. Hands are never sterile, i.e. have no living microorganism on them and this is why sterile disposable gloves are used for some procedures. *Candida albicans*, which often causes oral thrush in patients with advanced cancer can be spread to patients on the hands of nursing staff. Wearing sterile gloves when in contact with oral mucosa can prevent this spread.

Protective clothing is worn to prevent the transfer of microorganisms from room to room on clothing and to prevent the transfer of microorganisms from patient to nurse and *vice versa*. Such measures can make a significant difference especially when close contact with infectious patients is anticipated, e.g. lifting newborn babies (neonates). Impermeable, disposable plastic aprons changed after each dressing are better than cotton gowns which let microorganisms through the weave of the material, especially if it is wet.

Making sure that procedures such as bed-making and cleaning, which disperse microorganisms in the air, are not done immediately before dressing wounds can decrease airborne infection. It is also good practice to dress infected wounds last.

Care of central venous catheters

Central venous catheters (CVCs) can be surgically implanted in patients who need long-term intravenous therapy or can be inserted peripherally for short-term use. Almost 6000 patients a year in the UK acquire a catheter-related bloodstream infection (CR-BSI) associated with the insertion and maintenance of central venous catheters. These infections are among the most dangerous complications that can occur in a patient. The most commonly associated microorganism is *Staphylococcus epidermidis*. Infection is either from the hands of workers during care interventions or from microorganisms on the skin which contaminate the catheter during insertion (Fig. 7.11). Maximal sterile barrier precautions are essential when inserting CVCs and are more important than the environment, i.e. operating theatre or ward, while the catheter is inserted.

The recommendations from the guidelines to prevent healthcare associated infections suggest that the risk of infection can be minimised by:

- Selecting the right catheter for the patient, e.g. a single lumen catheter impregnated with an antimicrobial agent
- The best insertion site, e.g. the subclavian (shoulder) site is apparently preferable to the jugular (neck) or femoral (leg) site where possible
- Using aseptic technique during CVC placement, e.g. sterile gown, gloves and a large sterile drape
- The appropriate preparation of the insertion site, e.g. cleaning the skin with an alcoholic

chlorhexidine gluconate solution and allowing it to dry before insertion
- Effective care of the catheter and catheter site, e.g. disinfecting the external surfaces of the catheter and connecting ports, using a sterile gauze or transparent dressing to cover the site
- Adopting a CVC replacement strategy which looks at the method and frequency of replacement
- Not using antibiotics to decrease the risk of infection.

- Only using urinary catheters when there is no alternative procedure
- Selecting the smallest catheter which allows free urinary flow
- Using sterile equipment and aseptic technique for insertion
- Using a sterile closed system and preventing backflow of urine from drainage bags by positioning the bag below the level of the bladder and clamping the drainage bag tube when moving and handling patients.

Care of short-term indwelling urethral catheters in acute care

Urinary catheterisation is recognised as a major risk of HAIs. Between 20 and 30% of all catheterised patients develop bacteriuria (bacteria found in the urine). About 2% of these develop bacteraemia and around 22% of these die. It has also been shown that the risk of infection increases with the length of time that the catheter is in place. Clearly, good nursing practice is essential for this procedure.

The risk of infection can be minimised by:

Cleansing and disinfection

Cleansing is the process that removes visible dirt whereas disinfection will either kill or reduce the growth of microorganisms depending on the natural resistance of the microorganisms (Table 7.3). Disinfectants are generally harmful to the skin and protective clothing should be worn when they are used. Antiseptics are antimicrobial agents that decrease the growth of microorganisms on living tissues. Common examples of antiseptics are iodine and hydrogen peroxide.

Exercise 7.2

Make a list of the cleansers, disinfectants and antiseptics that you use at work or in your house. Can some be used as disinfectants and as an antiseptic? How can this be explained?

Cleansing and/or disinfection of equipment should be carried out between use with individual patients. Cleansing is needed for general soiling of items but disinfection is required for items that have been in contact with blood or body fluids or used with patients who have infections, e.g. methicillin resistant *Staphylococcus aureus* (MRSA), diarrhoea.

Cleansing should always precede disinfection because dirty equipment will protect any microroganisms which are present. Table 7.4 gives some examples of cleansing and disinfectant agents.

Disinfectants, which kill bacteria, are some-times referred to as bactericidal whereas those that only halt the growth are called bacteriostatic. A bactericidal disinfectant can be bacteriostatic when it is diluted. Therefore using disinfectants at the appropriate concentration is vital. Similarly, using the disinfectants for the correct period of time and ensuring that they are freshly prepared is essential for the procedure to be effective.

The most effective disinfectants are aldehydes, peroxides and halogen compounds but they are not suitable for use in every situation because of their harmful effects. These are all strong oxidising agents.

Table 7.4 Some examples of the use of disinfectant and cleansing agents

ITEM	ROUTINE CLEANSING	DISINFECTION
Patient wash bowls	General purpose liquid (GPL) detergent	0.1% hypochlorite solution
Suction machine jars	Disposable liners or liquid detergent	1% hypochlorite solution
Bedpan bases	GPL detergent	Hypochlorite disinfectant powder
Central lines	N/A	0.5% chlorhexidine in 70% industrial methylated spirit (IMS)
Bone marrow puncture	N/A	Aqueous or alcoholic Povidone–iodine® (10%)
Theatre trolleys	GPL detergent	70% isopropyl alcohol BP wipes
Lockers	GPL detergent	0.1% hypochlorite solution

Table 7.3 Resistance of microorganisms to disinfectants

Resistant microorganisms	Least resistant microorganisms
Bacterial endospores	Enveloped viruses
Non-enveloped viruses	Bacteria
	Fungi

Sterilisation

Sterilisation is a procedure that kills all living organisms including endospores and viruses. Autoclaving (which can be done in a pressure cooker) achieves sterilisation by using steam under pressure. It is commonly used for the sterilisation of general surgical instruments and anaesthetic masks. Higher temperatures are reached when steam is under pressure, e.g. 121°C at 108 kPa (15 psi) which will kill microorganisms in a shorter time than using heat at normal atmospheric pressure. Pre-packed sterile products, e.g. disposable syringes are sterilised at the factory using gamma-radiation for microorganism destruction.

Drug-resistant bacteria

Without antibiotics the world population would be lower and the job of the nurse more dangerous. But it is the very use of these 'miracle drugs' which has helped to create one of the major problems in hospitals today, antibiotic-resistant bacteria. or 'super-bugs'.

The dangers from drug-resistant bacteria have been well publicised in the media. Two groups, Gram-negative bacteria and Gram-positive Staphylococcus aureus are most frequently encountered. Figures from the Public Health Laboratory Service show that the proportion of Staphylococcus aureus strains sent to them which are resistant to antibiotics has increased from 1.5% in 1991 to more than 31% in 1997. Some strains, have even shown resistance to vancomycin, an antibiotic traditionally regarded as 'the last line of defence'.

Staphylococcus aureus is found on the skin and in the nose, therefore it can cause infections of wounds and indwelling devices. There are many different strains of methicillin or multiply resistant Staphylococcus aureus (MRSA) which vary in their ability to spread and cause infection. If a patient becomes infected then steps must be taken to prevent cross infection, e.g. closing the ward to new patients, screening of staff to see if they are infected. Thorough cleaning of the ward with disinfectants is necessary before new patients are admitted.

Gram-negative bacteria are part of the normal flora of the human gastrointestinal tract but can also cause upper respiratory

Table 7.5 Methods of transfer for antibiotic resistant plasmids

Method	Description	Bacteria
Transduction	Bacteriophage transfer of plasmids	*Staphylococcus aureus*
Conjugation	Transfer between donor male and recipient female bacteria of the same species via a conjugation tube formed from a sex pilus	Gram-negative bacteria
Transformation	DNA released from one bacterium is absorbed by another bacterium	*Streptococcus pneumoniae*

tract, urinary tract and wound infections. *Pseudomonas* spp. are particularly difficult to eliminate because there are few antibiotics that are effective against them. They are commonly identified in eye drops, tubing used for incubators and ventilators and soap solutions where warm moist conditions prevail. Development of antibiotic resistance in these microorganisms is problematic because the choice of available antibiotics becomes even more limited.

Gram-negative bacteraemia is a cause of septic shock which can occur before antibiotic sensitivities have been determined in the laboratory. This is very serious because if a multiply resistant bacterium is the cause, the first treatment given to the patient will probably be ineffective and patient death can result.

How do bacteria become resistant to drugs?

Growth of resistant microorganisms is not inhibited by the usual concentration of the antimicrobial agent. Resistance to drugs is expected because microorganisms adapt to their environment. Adaptation occurs by spontaneous mutations of DNA, which become apparent more quickly in bacteria because of their fast growth rates. This is called intrinsic resistance. Another type of intrinsic resistance is when the microorganism is naturally resistant to many antibiotics, e.g. *Pseudomonas aeruginosa*.

Intrinsic resistance is not the reason for the rapid spread of resistance in the bacterial population. This is dependent on the transfer of antibiotic resistant genes on plasmids by conjugation, transduction or less frequently transformation and is called acquired resistance (Table 7.5 and Fig. 7.12).

Transduction relies on bacteriophages. When the virus attacks the bacterium it makes the bacterium synthesise its nucleic acid and proteins which are then packaged into viral particles before their release when the cell is destroyed. Sometimes the packaging process is imperfect and a piece of DNA containing the antibiotic resistant genes, which could be a plasmid, is packaged into the bacteriophage proteins. This defective bacteriophage can attack another bacterial cell but will not destroy it because it contains bacterial DNA rather than viral nucleic acid. If the bacterial DNA contains antibiotic resistance gene(s) then the bacterium will become resistant and a multiply resistant bacterial population becomes established.

Conjugation in Gram-negative bacteria depends on the presence of a special plasmid called the F plasmid which codes for a pilus as well as other proteins. Cells which have a pilus (F+) can attach to a receptor on the surface of cells which do not have a pilus (F-). A conjugation tube is formed and a single strand of the plasmid DNA is transferred to the cell without the pilus. A complementary strand of DNA is synthesised in both cells so that each cell contains a double-stranded DNA plasmid called F+. Each of the F+ cells can transfer a copy of the plasmid to another F- cell so that the plasmid spreads rapidly throughout the population.

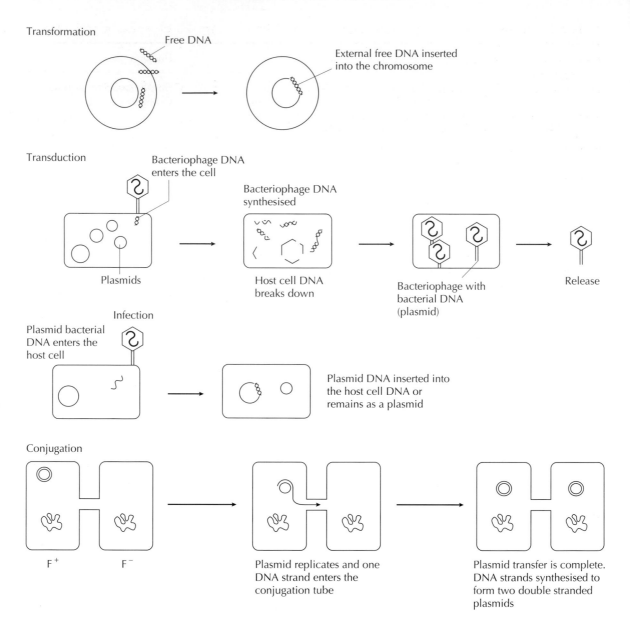

Fig. 7.12 Methods of antibiotic resistant plasmid transfer.

Transformation requires DNA which is outside the cell, i.e. the DNA has been released because the cell has died. The free DNA can be taken up by another cell of the same species and incorporated into the cell genome. It was first shown to be the means by which virulence could be acquired in *Streptococcus pneumo-* *niae* but is relatively insignificant in the spread of drug resistance.

What can be done?

There are four approaches that can be used to make the problem more manageable:

- Reduce the use of antibiotics
- Develop new therapeutic agents
- Ensure that patients take the full course of antibiotics
- Improve infection control.

The nurse can only be truly active in the last of these methods. Recognition of your role in preventing infections and compliance with procedures is key to reducing the transmission of microorganisms.

Summary

- Bacterial (prokaryote) cells have a different structure from human (eukaryote) cells
- Growth of bacteria is very rapid
- Bacteria can be divided into two groups by the Gram stain (Gram-positive, purple and Gram-negative, pink)
- Hospital acquired infection (HAI) can be minimised by effective personal hygiene and care of catheters
- Methods used to cleanse, disinfect and sterilise are dependent on the probable contaminating microorganisms and the particular situation

- The rapid spread of antibiotic resistance is achieved by plasmid transfer.

Review questions

7.1. What are the differences between the growth of a bacterium, a virus, and a yeast?

7.2. Distinguish between:
 (a) cross infection and self infection
 (b) sterilisation and disinfection.

7.3. Why is hand washing important?

7.4. Which groups of bacteria are associated with drug resistance?

7.5. How are bacteria transmitted to pieces of equipment and what method could you use to remove them?

Further reading

Journal of Hospital Infection (2001). **47 (Supplement)**: S29–S47.

Stucke, V. (1998). *Microbiology for Nurses* (7th edn). Baillière Tindall, London.

Gould, D. and Brooker, C. (2000). *Applied Microbiology for Nurses*. Macmillan Press Ltd, London.

Chapter Eight
IMMUNOLOGY

Learning objectives

By the end of this chapter the reader will be able to:
- Review the defence mechanisms of the body to infection
- Distinguish between innate and adaptive immunity
- Describe specific immune responses against intracellular and extracellular pathogens
- Explain how the immune system has been used for vaccination and rapid diagnostic tests.

Introduction

Most of the time you are healthy and free from infection. When you do get an infection you will normally recover because your body recognises the microorganism as 'foreign' and works to remove or destroy it. Sometimes the immune system can produce unwanted effects (hypersensitivity – graft rejection and asthma) or may not work very well at all due to hereditary defects or specific infections.

This chapter looks at the way the immune system works and how it has been exploited to produce vaccines giving us protection against major pathogens.

The immune system

The immune system is made up of all the cells, tissues and organs required for an immune response. Its function is to protect us from pathogens and destroy cells which are no longer recognised as 'self'. If the system breaks down, auto immune disease, immunodeficiency or allergic diseases can be the result.

Surface barriers

The immune system allows recovery from infections caused by microorganisms which have invaded the surface barriers of the body (Table 8.1). Hospital patients are more likely to be at risk of invasion because their illness or treatment breaks down their normal defence mechanisms. Examples include burns, urinary catheterisation, neutropenia (low neutrophil/white blood cell count), lack of normal bacterial flora and malnutrition in either postoperative patients or patients who are in intensive care.

The first line of defence for the body is the skin (surface barrier). If this is overcome or bypassed the inflammatory response is triggered.

The inflammatory response

The most visible sign of your immune system working is the redness, swelling and pain that you see and/or feel when injured or invaded by foreign materials. This reaction is called the inflammatory response.

The signs are caused by:

Table 8.1 Surface barriers of the body

Barrier	Mechanism
Skin	Physical barrier
Normal bacterial flora (commensals)	Competes effectively with pathogens on skin, in the intestines, vagina and upper respiratory tract
Lysozyme in tears, body secretions (not urine) and tissues	Breaks down the cell wall of bacteria
pH	Low pH in stomach and vagina discourages bacterial growth
Mucous membranes	Traps microorganisms and stops them sticking to epithelial cells

- Dilation of the blood vessels, which increases blood flow so that more blood reaches the affected area
- Increased capillary permeability, which allows large molecules of the immune system and phagocytes to migrate into the tissues
- Chemicals, such as histamine and lymphokines that are released from damaged cells
- The accumulation of inflammatory fluids that ooze into a confined space, resulting in increased pressure.

These effects localise the area, dilute the irritants and eliminate them by phagocytosis. Inflammatory conditions are common e.g. colitis, meningitis, pneumonia and pleurisy. Sometimes the inflammatory response lasts too long and can result in tissue death, e.g. gangrene and tuberculosis.

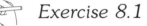

Exercise 8.1

Think of as many inflammatory conditions as you can. Hint: most of them end in 'itis'.

Innate and adaptive immunity

The immune system can distinguish between its own 'self' cells and components and 'foreign' substances, which are called antigens. The immune response describes the recognition of the antigen and its elimination.

There are two functional parts to the immune system, the innate system, which acts first against any antigen and an adaptive system which is activated when the innate system fails. Both systems will then work together.

The adaptive response is specific to a particular antigen and your immune system will remember it. This means that once you have successfully activated an immune response against an antigen you will be able to respond to it more quickly if you are exposed to it a second time. Both the innate and adaptive systems depend on cells and soluble components to work (Table 8.2).

White blood cells of the immune system

White blood cells (WBCs) are our main defence against microorganisms. They have to cross the blood vessel walls to reach the tissues that have been infected with microorganisms. They can be divided into two groups based on their

Table 8.2 Components of the immune system

	Cells	Soluble factors
Innate immunity	Phagocytes	Complement, lysozyme
Adaptive immunity	Natural killer cells (NK)	Interferon Antibodies
	T and B cells (lymphocytes)	

Table 8.3 Cells of the immune system

Cell type	Function
Lymphocytes:	
1. B lymphocytes (B-cells)	Adaptive immunity (antibody production)
2. T lymphocytes (T-cells)*	Adaptive immunity (destruction of intracellular pathogens)
3. Natural killer cells	Innate immunity (cytotoxic, kill foreign cells)
Polymorphonuclear phagocytes:	
1. Neutrophils	Phagocytosis
2. Eosinophils, basophils	Involved in allergic reactions and parasite destruction
Mononuclear phagocytes:	
1. Monocytes (differentiate into macrophages in the tissues)	Phagocytosis of intracellular microorganisms, e.g. mycobacteria
2. Macrophages	Assist in immune response, phagocytosis

*T-cells can be further divided by their activity into helper, suppressor, cytotoxic and memory cells.

function. One group, the phagocytes, engulf the invading substances and destroy them. The other group, the lymphocytes, are vital for long-term defence. However phagocytes and lymphocytes can work together, particularly to generate adaptive immune responses. The types and functions of some of the cells are shown in Table 8.3.

Soluble factors of the immune system

There are many different soluble factors involved in the immune response. Some are produced by lymphocytes, e.g. antibodies and cytokines and others are present in the blood serum. Their functions are shown in Table 8.4.

Complement is a series of about 20 serum proteins which are activated either by antigen/antibody complexes in adaptive immunity or microorganisms in innate immunity. Activation of the first component then activates the next so that the sequence of events is like a cascade.

Different parts of the cascade result in three main effects:

- More effective phagocytosis (opsonisation) because complement covers immune complexes and microorganisms so that phagocytes with complement receptors can bind efficiently to them
- Cell lysis (disruption)
- Phagocyte activation.

Cytokines are the molecules which act as messengers between cells; lymphokines are therefore cytokines, which communicate with lymphocytes.

Antibodies or immunoglobulins (Ig) are produced from plasma cells (differentiated B lym-

Table 8.4 Soluble factors of the immune system

Component	Function
Cytokines:	
1. Interferons	Virus resistance
2. Interleukins	Direct the division and differentiation of cells
3. Colony stimulating factors	Division and differentiation of bone marrow cells
Complement	Control of inflammation
C-reactive protein	Activates complement by binding to bacteria
Antibodies	Neutralisation of antigens

phocytes). All antibodies have the same basic structure (Fig. 8.1) which allows them to bind with antigens, phagocytes and complement. However because all antigens are different, the antigen binding site is made up of different amino acids (the variable region). This allows a specific antibody to be produced against each of the many antigens to which we are exposed.

Antibody types

There are five classes of antibody or immunoglobulin molecules, each of which have a different function. IgG is the most common and can cross the placenta to provide protection for the newborn. IgM is made up of five basic units and is the first line of attack for bacteria. IgA is present in secretions, e.g. saliva, colostrum, milk and tracheobronchial secretions. IgD is found on the surface of B-cells but in very low concentrations in human serum, its function is unclear and IgE is associated with allergies, e.g. asthma. The relative amounts of the immunoglobin classes are shown in Table 8.5.

Immune system structure

The immune system has a constant watching role and the components must be ready and able to reach the affected area quickly if they are to be effective. The lymphoid system makes

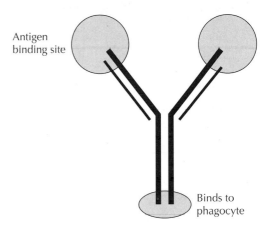

Fig. 8.1 Antibody structure.

Table 8.5 Immunoglobulin classes in human serum

Immunoglobulin (Ig) type	% of total Ig in human serum
IgG	70–75
IgM	10
IgA	15–20
IgD	>1
IgE	Scarce

up the tissues and cells needed for the immune response. The tissues involved are shown in Fig. 8.2.

The major sites of lymphocyte production are the bone marrow and thymus. The spleen,

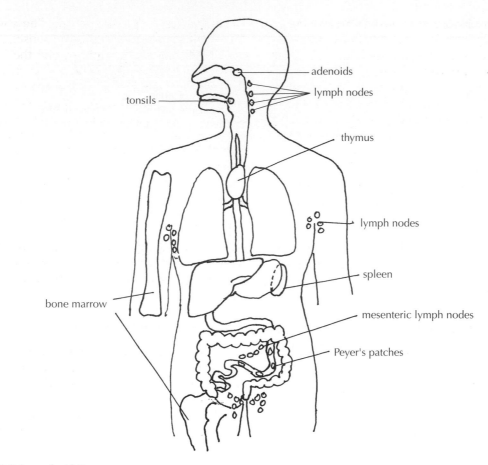

Fig. 8.2 Lymphoid tissues.

lymph nodes and mucosa-associated tissues, e.g. tonsils (peripheral organs and tissues) are the sites where cells of the immune response react with the antigen. The spleen is particularly good at filtering out microorganisms. If the spleen is removed the immune system is considerably less effective.

The lymphocytes move from their site of production to the peripheral tissues via the blood and lymphatic system (a network of small channels all over the body). About 1–2% of the lymphocytes recirculate each hour but if an antigen is recognised then circulation is stopped so that the antigen-sensitised cells can be localised in the lymph nodes where the antigen is first seen.

This means that a good immune response can be achieved quickly.

Antigen recognition

It has already been said that recognition of an antigen (foreign substance) is the first step in activating the immune system. This means that it must recognise the cells which belong to the body so that they are not destroyed. All cells are labelled, so that this is possible, with a protein marker called the major histocompatibility complex (MHC). There are two MHC sets, Class I and Class II.

When a microorganism first enters the body it is phagocytosed by macrophages because it is not recognised as a normal body cell. It is destroyed or 'processed' so that peptide fragments of the antigen appear on the surface of the cell with the MHC molecules. The macrophage is then called an antigen presenting cell (APC). This term can be used for any cell, which has a processed antigen sticking out from its surface. It includes new B-cells that have antibody molecules all over their surface membrane which bind specifically to a microorganism. The microorganism is then taken into the cell and processed. APCs present the antigen with either MHC Class I or Class II proteins, which determines the type of T-cell that they react with.

Antibody production

Antibodies are produced by B-cells that are stimulated to divide by binding to an antigen. For most antigens, the B-cell cannot divide without signals from the T-helper cell (Th) which responds to an APC with the same processed antigen (Fig. 8.3). A positive reaction causes the

T cells to multiply (proliferate) and differentiate. The T-helper cells react with the sensitised B-cell by recognising the antigen and the MHC Class II molecules. They produce interleukins (ILs) which result in the production of large numbers of effector B-cells (plasma cells) that secrete antibodies specific to the original antigen. A small number of B and T memory cells are also synthesised for a future secondary response (Fig. 8.3).

When the antigen has been eliminated the antibodies will not be needed any more and their synthesis is stopped by a different type of T-cell called T supressor cells. Not all the antibodies will be used up, which means that some will be circulating in the blood. This is very useful for diagnosing viral diseases, e.g. hepatitis.

Immune response time

If the antigen is new, the time taken for antibodies to appear in the blood will be longer (primary immune response) than if the antigen has been seen before (secondary response) (Fig. 8.4). The secondary response is the basis of vaccination booster schedules.

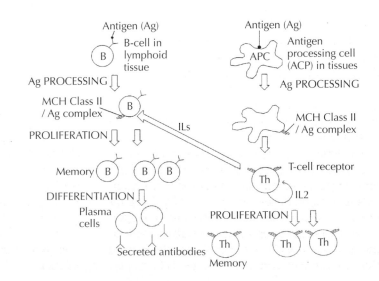

Fig. 8.3 Antibody production.

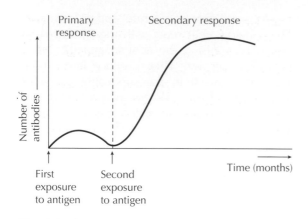

Fig. 8.4 The immune response.

Cell-mediated immune response

Antibodies are effective against pathogens and toxins which are extracellular, but they cannot bind to intracellular pathogens, e.g. viruses and toxins. Fortunately another response from the immune system is possible which only involves T-cells, the cell-mediated immune response (Fig. 8.5). Not only is this effective against intracellular pathogens but it will also recognise abnormal cells, e.g. cancer cells and grafted organ tissue cells. For organ transplant patients it is therefore vital that good tissue matches are made and that drugs are given which suppress the immune response so that the organ is not rejected. The T-cells also increase a number of other cells, e.g. macrophages, which enhance the removal of infected cells. In chronic inflammatory conditions, e.g. tuberculosis, granulomas (collections of fused macrophages, giant cells, epithelial and T-cells) form which calcify leading to a loss of function of the tissue.

T-cells mature in the thymus where they differentiate into T-helper and cytotoxic T-cells and synthesise receptors for one specific antigen, i.e. each T-cell will respond to a different antigen. These new/naive T-cells enter the bloodstream and remain inactive until they meet an antigen-presenting cell with an antigen MHC Class I or Class II complex on its surface that it can recognise.

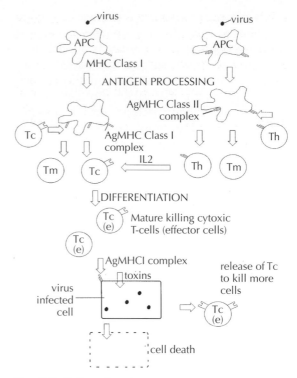

Fig. 8.5 Cell-mediated response.

Recognition of the complex stimulates the appropriate T-cell (Th/MHC Class II, Tc/MHC Class I) to divide and produce a population or clone of cells, which will react with the same antigen MHC complex. Helped by the T-helper cells, which produce interleukins, a clone of cytoxic T-cells differentiates into effector and memory cells that all respond to the same antigen. Interaction with an infected or 'foreign' cell activates the cytotoxic T-cell to kill it by punching holes in the plasma membrane and secreting toxins into it. The cytotoxic T-cell is then free to attack another cell.

Results of the adaptive immune responses

The adaptive immune processes have two effects:

- Antibodies neutralise the antigen to make it ineffective, activate complement and help in the inflammatory response
- Cytotoxic T-cells kill 'foreign' cells.

The key points of adaptive immunity are that it is specific to a particular antigen and that the antigen is remembered. This enables the body to respond to the same antigen when it is seen again.

Defective immune responses

Sometimes the immune system does not work properly; probably the example with which you are most familiar is a hypersensitivity reaction, where the immune response is too great. These are characterised by an immediate or delayed inflammatory reaction to an antigen, that is normally harmless. Common examples of such antigens are antibiotics, cosmetics, foods (such as nuts) and sticking plasters.

People, who are hypersensitive or 'allergic', synthesise IgE every time they are exposed to the allergen, which binds to the surface of white blood cells called mast cells. The next exposure to the antigen means that the allergen binds to the IgE on the mast cell surface which triggers the release of histamine and other chemicals from the mast cell. This causes the muscles in the airways to contract and the production of mucus that can result in an asthma attack.

Rarely, the inflammatory reaction spreads very rapidly, the airways constrict, blood pressure drops and circulatory collapse follows. Typically this kind of reaction is seen in people who are allergic to wasp and bee stings and is referred to as anaphylactic shock.

Desensitisation to antigens

One approach to treating people who are hypersensitive is to desensitise them by giving low doses of the antigen so that only IgG rather than IgE is produced. By increasing the concentration of antigen given over a period of time the concentration of circulating IgG is increased. When the antigen is next encountered IgG binds to it which decreases the amount of antigen that can bind to IgE on the surface of the mast cells, effectively preventing a hypersensitive reaction (inflammatory response).

Immune incompetence

People can be born with immunodeficient systems (defects in antibody production or T-cell function) or patients can become immunodeficient from infections such as AIDS (acquired immunodeficiency syndrome), which attacks the T-helper cell population, and haematological malignancies. Alternatively, patients can be immunosuppressed by drugs, e.g. renal transplant patients, or cancer patients treated with cytotoxic drugs that are capable of destroying cells. Obviously all these people are susceptible to infections which would not normally be life threatening. Nursing care of these patients must be particularly rigorous.

Autoimmune diseases

In autoimmune diseases the immune system no longer recognises its own cells and starts to attack them. Two relatively common diseases of this type are rheumatoid arthritis and systemic lupus erythematosus (SLE). Rheumatoid arthritis affects the membranes of the joints starting in the small joints of the hands and feet. Affected people have high levels of an antibody (rheumatoid factor), which binds to IgG molecules like an antigen. The complexes then accumulate on the membranes of the joints, which triggers a chronic inflammatory response eventually immobilising the joint. In SLE, the patients develop antibodies to their DNA and the complexes accumulate in the blood vessels, joints and kidneys. Why autoimmune responses begin remains unexplained and effective treatment is unlikely until this process is understood.

Applications of the immune system

We already know that antibodies are made in response to antigens. We have made use of this knowledge by making the body produce antibodies against diseases (active immunity) or giving antibodies to protect us from disease (passive immunity). More recently we have been able to develop a special type of antibody called monoclonal antibodies that are produced from cells grown in culture. Monoclonal antibodies are identical and highly specific; they have been used very successfully to improve diagnostic techniques and have the potential to be used for large-scale treatment.

Active immunisation

Vaccines are given to effect active immunity in an individual by stimulating antibody production, which can last for years. You will be familiar with immunisation schedules for children (Table 8.6) or having vaccinations before you visit certain countries. Effective immunisation programmes can prevent infectious diseases or control their spread. Some diseases, such as smallpox, have been eliminated world wide by vaccination. A more recent example is the success of meningitis C vaccination which has significantly decreased the incidence of the disease.

Four types of vaccine

There are four types of vaccine shown in Table 8.6. Generally, live, attenuated or non-virulent strains of a pathogen are used for protection against viruses and inactivated bacteria are used for bacterial diseases. However, there are exceptions – Bacillus Calmette-Guérin (BCG) vaccine for tuberculosis is a live, attenuated form and influenza is a killed virus.

The important difference is that live, attenuated strains replicate whereas inactivated strains do not. This means that immunity from live vaccines is longer lasting and usually achieved with a single dose but inactivated vaccines often require boosters and only last for months.

An acellular vaccine for pertussis protection (whooping cough) has been introduced from November 2001 as part of the pre-school booster vaccine (OTaP). Acellular vaccines use a small part of the microorganisms e.g. capsule polysaccharides to raise an antibody response. Whole cell pertussis vaccine cannot be used as a booster because it gives an increased rate of reaction in older children.

Table 8.6 Immunisation schedule for children

Vaccine	Type	Age when given
Diphtheria/tetanus/whole cell pertussis (OTwP)	Toxoid/inactivated bacteria	First year
Polio	Live, attenuated virus	First year
Haemophilus influenzae, type B (HiB) (Given as DTwP-Hib)	Capsular polysaccharide	First year
Measles/Mumps/Rubella (MMR)	Live, attenuated virus	Second year
Diphtheria/Tetanus/Acellular pertussis (OTaP) booster	Inactivated bacteria/toxin	5 years
Polio booster	Live, attenuated virus	5 years
Bacillus Calmette-Guérin (BCG)	Live, attenuated bacteria	10–14 years
Meningitis C (MenC)	Capsular polysaccharide conjugate	Under 18 years

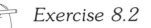

Exercise 8.2

A mother asks you why her child should be immunised when most of the diseases occur only rarely. How would you respond to her question?

Vaccines are not available for all diseases

Some diseases are not easily controlled by vaccination, e.g. cholera. The vaccine is made from killed bacteria although new cholera vaccines are being developed. An enterotoxin causes the typical diarrhoea of cholera and neither the enterotoxin nor the bacteria are released into the bloodstream. Therefore although circulating antibodies to the bacteria are produced from the vaccine by an immune response, they have to reach the intestinal tissue that is infected by the bacteria. This makes the vaccine relatively ineffective because only a small number of antibodies will make contact with the bacteria.

Another example is viral influenza. The influenza virus is able to mutate (change) easily, so the vaccine has to be reviewed each year to ensure that the strains used for the vaccination programme will give the best protection to 'at risk' groups. In 2001, two strains of Influenza A (H3N2 and H1N1) and Influenza B (Sichuan) were used.

Activity

Make a list of diseases which have no effective vaccines, e.g. AIDS, malaria and gonorrhoea. See if you can find the reason(s) for this.

Passive immunisation

Passive immunisation gives immediate protection but only lasts for a few weeks. Injections of pooled plasma, containing antibodies or immunoglobulins against the disease, are given to those at risk. Antiserum (plasma containing antibodies from animals) is rarely given now because side-effects frequently result.

Immunoglobulins are of two types, human normal immunoglobulin (HNIG) and specific immunoglobulins. HNIG is used for the protection of hepatitis A virus, measles and rubella. Specific immunoglobulins are shown in Table 8.7.

Antibodies used for treatment and diagnostic tests

An exciting development, which can be exploited in many areas today, is the production of monoclonal antibodies. These are antibodies that are produced in cell culture and only respond to one part of an antigen. All the antibodies are identical so a very specific and effective reaction is possible. The reaction can be 'seen' by labelling the antibody with a tag such as a radioactive isotope or fluorescent dye. Some examples of their potential use relevant to patient health are: tracking foreign materials, e.g. cancer cells; allowing better tissue typing prior to organ transplants and rapid diagnostic testing, e.g. pregnancy kits and blood typing.

Table 8.7 Specific immunolobulins used for passive immunisation

Specific immunoglobulin	Use
Hepatitis B immunoglobulin (HBIG)	Infants born to infected mothers, personnel working with the virus
Tetanus immunoglobulin (HTIG)	Management of tetanus-prone wounds
Varicella-zoster immunoglobulin (VZIG)	Women exposed to chickenpox during pregnancy, immunosupressed patients

Magic bullets

If antibodies are tagged with a chemical that can destroy the cell with which it reacts it is theoretically possible to eliminate all the cells which react with the antibody. This approach is being researched to provide a treatment for cancer. For example, radioactive isotopes, e.g. ^{131}I, tagged to antibodies could bind to tumour cells and destroy them. The radioactive isotope could also be transmitted to cells to which the antibody has not bound, thereby increasing the radioactive dose. Antibodies to tumour cells bound to cytotoxic drugs are also being investigated.

Organ transplants

Monoclonal antibodies have improved the success of organ transplants in two ways. Firstly, better matching of donor and recipient tissue types before organ transplants is possible. Secondly, by preventing cytotoxic T-cells binding to the donor organ, which would destroy it. Treating the patient with this antibody has improved the success rate of kidney transplant operations by 90%.

Dipsticks/strips

In immunological diagnostic tests, antibodies are labelled so that it is easy to see a test result. A good example is preganancy-testing kits. In these tests antibodies are attached to coloured latex particles, which respond to human chorionic gonadotrophin (hCG) found in the urine of pregnant women. The test strip has mobile antibodies at the bottom and immobilised antibodies (ones which cannot move) in two different places further up the strip.

When the strip is placed in a urine sample the mobile antibodies attached to coloured latex particles react with the hormone and diffuse up the strip until they reach the first band of immobilised antibodies that bind to hCG/mobile antibody complex. This results in a coloured band forming indicating a positive test. If the woman is not pregnant there will be no reaction. The urine continues to move up the strip to the higher band where a second band of antibodies are immobilised. These bind to the mobile antibodies alone. A single coloured band at the higher level indicates a negative test and shows that the test has worked. Two coloured bands indicate a positive test (Fig. 8.6).

Blood typing

Blood is classified into four main groups by the type of antigens on the surface of red blood cells, the antibodies circulating in the plasma and the presence or absence of the Rhesus (D) antigen. The genes, which code for the antigens, have three alleles A, B and O. A and B are co-dominant and can appear together, but when A or B is paired with O antigen, the O phenotype is not expressed (Table 8.8).

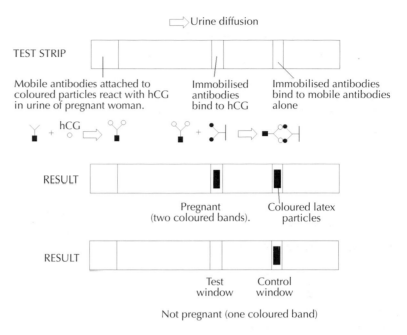

Fig. 8.6 Strip used for pregnancy testing.

Table 8.8 Human blood groups

Genotype	Phenotype	% population	AB in plasma	Phenotype of blood which can be received
$I^I I^I$	O	45	A, B	O
$I^A I^A$ or $I^A I^I$	A	40	B	A and O
$I^B I^B$ or $I^B I^I$	B	10	A	B and O
$I^A I^B$	AB	5	None	Any

⧖⧗ *Activity*

Perhaps you are a blood donor and know your blood type. Can you work out the possible blood type of your parents? Could you give them blood?

Blood type can be determined by mixing specific antibodies with the blood sample. So if you have blood group A, the cells will have the A antigen and will react with anti-A antibodies. This is seen as clumping or agglutination of the blood cells indicating a positive reaction. Testing the same blood with anti-B antigen antibodies would not result in agglutination showing that the blood was not type B.

It is vital to know the blood group of a patient if they are likely to need a blood transfusion. Mixing incompatible blood together will agglutinate the donor red blood cells and then cause them to burst (haemolyse) (Fig. 8.7). The reaction can be fatal.

The other major antigen that is important in blood grouping is the Rhesus antigen or D antigen. About 85% of the population is Rhesus

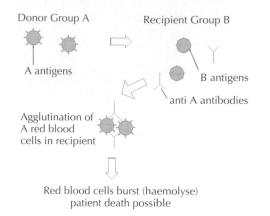

Fig. 8.7 Agglutination of blood cells.

positive. The antigen was first found in monkeys, hence the name. If you are Rhesus positive you have the antigen on your red blood cells but no circulating Rh antibodies. However if you are Rhesus negative, with no antigen on your red blood cells, and receive some positive blood you will produce antibodies to it.

This becomes significant in Rhesus negative women during pregnancy who may have a Rhesus positive fetus. When the baby is born she may receive some fetal blood cells to which she will produce antibodies. If her next baby is Rhesus positive, her antibodies will destroy the blood of the baby (Haemolytic disease of the newborn). Today, Rhesus negative mothers are given an antibody D injection immediately after birth, which destroys any Rhesus positive cells from the baby in the mother's circulation. This means that the next child will not be affected. The dose of injected antibody is too small to have any effect on future pregnancies.

Summary

- Our immune system is vital to keep us free from infection
- Infections result when the surface barriers of the body are penetrated
- Immunity can be divided into innate or non-specific immunity and adaptive or specific immunity but the systems work together
- Specific immunity has different mechanisms for extracellular pathogens (antibodies) and intracellular pathogens (cellular immunity)
- The immune system does not always function properly, e.g. allergies and autoimmune diseases
- The specific antibody response has been exploited to make vaccines allowing people to be protected against major pathogens
- Monoclonal antibodies are being used for the development of diagnostic tests and cancer therapy.

Review questions

8.1. How does the structure of an antibody help to ensure the efficient removal of an antigen?

8.2. Explain why people with AIDS are vulnerable to infections.

8.3. What are the characteristics of adaptive immunity?

8.4. Define the term cytokine.

8.5. What are the characteristics of the inflammatory response?

8.6. How does immunisation with a vaccine give protection against disease?

Further reading

Playfair, J.H.L. & Chain, B.M. (2001). *Immunology at a Glance* (7th edn). Blackwell Science Ltd, Oxford.

Roitt, I.M. & Delves, P.J. (2001). Roitt's Essential Immunology (10th edn.). Blackwell Science Ltd, Oxford.

Chapter Nine
FLUIDS – LIQUIDS AND GASES

Learning objectives

By the end of the chapter the reader will be able to:
- Define the term pressure and list its units
- State Pascal's principle
- Describe factors that affect blood flow in the body
- Explain the procedure for measuring blood pressure
- State the gas laws – Boyle's, Henry's & Dalton's
- Describe the process of breathing by applying Boyle's Law
- Explain how gases are exchanged in the body applying Dalton's and Henry's laws
- Describe oxygen therapy
- Explain how a nebuliser works.

Introduction

The body needs a continuous supply of the gas oxygen. Oxygen is used in the cells for respiration which results in the waste product carbon dioxide. We can live without food and water for days, but without oxygen our cells would starve and die within minutes. Also, the carbon dioxide produced is toxic to the body in high concentrations. Gases, therefore, need to move around and in and out of the body.

Blood is the only tissue in the body that is a fluid. It transports both oxygen and nutrients to the tissues and removes their waste products such as carbon dioxide. Blood is probably examined more often in hospital laboratories than any other tissue from the body. Liquids and gases flow, so they are both fluids in contrast with solids which are rigid.

Pressure

Scientists define pressure as the force per unit area:

$$\text{Pressure} = \frac{\text{Force}}{\text{Area}}$$

The greater the area over which a force acts, the less the pressure. This is why wearing skis prevents you sinking into soft snow since your weight is spread over a large area.

Injecting liquid from different size syringes can also be used to illustrate the concept of pressure. Assuming that the force of the thumb is the same, a narrow syringe generates a much larger pressure than a wider syringe (Fig. 9.1). Therefore using small syringes to give injections can result in large pressures and can cause damage to tissue and veins.

Atmospheric pressure

The air forming the earth's atmosphere stretches upwards for miles. The force of gravity on the air molecules gives rise to atmospheric pressure. We do not normally feel atmospheric pressure because the pressure inside our bodies is almost the same as the pressure outside.

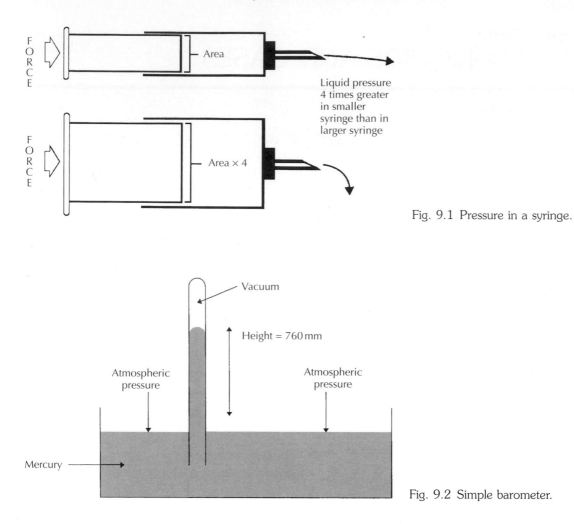

Fig. 9.1 Pressure in a syringe.

Fig. 9.2 Simple barometer.

In the 17th century Torricelli measured atmospheric pressure using a simple manometer (Fig. 9.2). In his experiment Torricelli filled a tube with mercury and inverted it into a bowl of mercury. When inverted the column of mercury sank, creating a near vacuum (a space from which all the air has been drawn) at the top of the tube, the column was approximately 760 mm above the level of the mercury in the bowl. It was prevented from falling any further by atmospheric pressure, which presses on the mercury in the bowl, in effect holding the column up. He found that the exact height of the mercury column depended on location and

the weather. Torricelli used millimetres (mm) to measure the height of the column and since he used mercury (Hg), the unit mmHg is used for pressure.

Atmospheric pressure (as any other pressure) can move fluids from areas of high pressure to areas of low pressure and in the clinical area you will use this to fill a hypodermic syringe, siphon and suction (Fig. 9.3).

In clinical practice the terms 'negative' and 'positive' pressures are commonly used especially in the respiratory system. A positive pressure is any pressure above atmospheric pressure, e.g. 770 mmHg or +10 mmHg is a positive

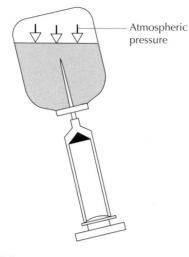

Atmospheric pressure

Fig. 9.3 Filling a syringe.

pressure. Any pressure below atmospheric pressure is a negative pressure, e.g. 755 mmHg or –5 mmHg.

Units of pressure

The SI unit of pressure is the Pascal (Pa). A Pascal is the pressure of one Newton acting over an area of one square metre. It is quite a small pressure – e.g. an apple in your hand exerts about 1000 Pascals. We therefore use the kilopascal (kPa). 1000 Pa = 1 kPa.

There are several units of pressure and you will encounter them all in clinical practice. Table 9.1 summarises some pressure units and where you will encounter them.

One unit can be readily converted into another by using the following conversion factors.

Conversion factors

$$1\,kPa = 7.5\,mmHg = 10.2\,cmH_2O$$

$$14.5\,lb\,inch^{-2} = 1\,bar = 750\,mmHg$$

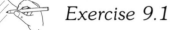

Exercise 9.1

a) Convert the following to kilopascals:
    i) 760 mmHg   ii) 120 mmHg
b) Convert the following to cmH$_2$O
    i) 0.5 kPas   ii) 760 mmHg

Liquids

Liquids have a fixed volume but their shape depends on the container. In the same way as the force of gravity on air results in atmospheric pressure, so the force of gravity on liquids gives rise to pressure within them.

Pascal's principle

Pascal's principle states that *in an enclosed liquid, pressure acts in all directions* and that *any change in pressure is transmitted equally to every part of the liquid*. A number of body cavities contain fluid, the eye being one (Fig. 9.4). The fluid inside the eye protects the retina. However, if a severe blow is applied to the cornea then this pressure will be transmitted into the interior of the eye and to the retina and optical nerve. Glaucoma is a condition that involves a build-up of pressure in the eye due to the accumulation of fluid which results from the poor drainage of the aqueous humour. This increased pressure compresses

Special Senses

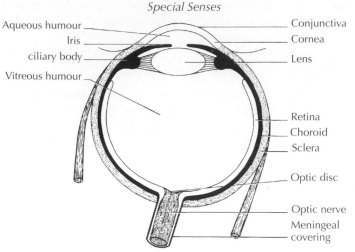

Aqueous humour
Iris
ciliary body
Vitreous humour

Conjunctiva
Cornea
Lens

Retina
Choroid
Sclera

Optic disc

Optic nerve
Meningeal covering

Fig. 9.4 Diagram of the eye.

Table 9.1 Pressure units

Unit	Notes
Pascal (Pa)/kilopascal (kPa)	blood gases
mmHg	arterial blood pressure, weather maps
cmH$_2$O	central venous pressure
Atmosphere (Atm)	gas cylinders, autoclaves
Bar	gas cylinders, oil pressure in cars
Torr (1 Torr = 1 mmHg)	vacuum gauges
lb inch^{-2} (psi)	gas cylinders, tyre pressure for cars

the retina and optic nerve leading to blindness if untreated.

Another body cavity containing fluid is the uterus (womb) during pregnancy, this is amniotic fluid. Any increase in pressure in any part of the fluid is transmitted to the fetus. The advantage of this is that any blow to the uterus is distributed uniformly through the fluid, so the fetus is protected.

Pressure in liquids

The pressure exerted by a column of a liquid is proportional to the height of the column and the density of the liquid. Let us look at these two factors more closely:

- **Height** – If the height of an intravenous infusion (IV) bag is raised relative to the patient the flow rate of the fluid will increase. For intravenous infusions a prescribed volume of fluid needs to be infused in a set time. However patients move and may change their position from supine (lying down) to walking – this will change the rate of delivery of the fluid. Due to this the flow rate needs to be checked continually (see Fig. 9.5).
- **Density** – the densities of liquids vary. Mercury is 13.5 times heavier than water, therefore if you had columns of both, each the same height, the column of mercury would exert 13.5 times more pressure than that of water.

Blood – pressure, resistance and flow

Blood is simply a fluid that flows through containers or vessels and its movement, like any other fluid, is governed by basic principles.

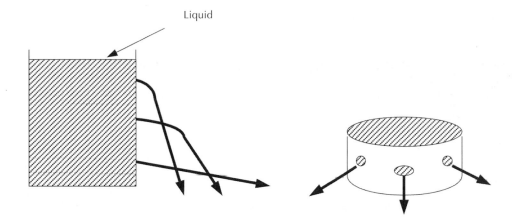

Pressure in a liquid increases with depth – the liquid flows out fastest from the bottom hole

Pressure at one depth acts equally in all directions so liquid flow is equal from all holes

Fig. 9.5 Liquids in containers.

Pressure

All fluids in containers exert a pressure. Hydrostatic pressure is the force that a liquid exerts against the wall of a container. The pressure that the blood exerts in the circulatory or vascular system on the blood vessel walls is known as blood pressure – blood pressure is therefore a hydrostatic pressure.

The pressure a fluid column exerts depends on its height. Blood is a fluid and therefore hydrostatic effects means that blood pressure will vary depending on the location at which blood pressure is measured (Fig. 9.6). Due to this a standard reference point is needed, this is taken as the heart.

Pascal's principle can also be applied to blood. If a blood vessel has a weak spot any increase in blood pressure inside the blood vessel is transmitted equally in all directions. If the pressure gets big enough the wall of the vessel can burst. Fluids flow down a pressure gradient – that is from an area of high pressure to an area of low pressure. It is the difference in pressure that is important, not the actual values of pressure.

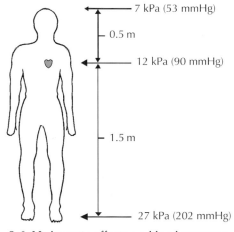

7 kPa (53 mmHg)

0.5 m

12 kPa (90 mmHg)

1.5 m

27 kPa (202 mmHg)

Fig. 9.6 Hydrostatic effects on blood pressure.

There is a large pressure gradient in the circulatory system. The pressure in the aorta is approximately 100 mmHg since blood is pumped directly into it. The pressure falls slowly but progressively through the circulatory system to 0 mmHg at the right atrium. This drop in pressure is due to resistance.

Measurement of arterial blood pressure

Normally when nurses refer to blood pressure they mean the arterial blood pressure. A single heart beat consists of a wave of contraction, called systole, followed by a relaxation phase called diastole. Thus the blood pressure in the major arteries rises and falls as the heart contracts and relaxes. The maximum pressure, which occurs after contraction of the ventricles is called the systolic pressure. The minimum pressure is known as the diastolic pressure and occurs when arterial pressure has dropped before the next contraction of the ventricles. The values of blood pressure are recorded as fractions, e.g. 120/80. The systolic pressure is the top figure and the diastolic pressure is the bottom figure. The contraction and relaxation of the heart are accompanied by sounds. In the arteries these can be heard by listening with a stethoscope placed over the brachial artery of the arm, whilst using a sphygmomanometer. These sounds are named after the Russian surgeon, Dr Nicholai Korotkov, who developed this procedure (Fig. 9.7). The origin of the sounds is thought to be due to turbulent flow.

Using the sphygmomanometer

By using a sphygmomanometer and a stethoscope, arterial blood pressure can be measured accurately by a non-invasive method (Fig. 9.8).

- Sit the patient comfortably, in a quiet environment
- Make sure their arm is resting at heart level
- Locate the brachial artery by palpitation
- Assess the maximal inflation level by inflating the cuff and palpating the radial pulse at the same time; the level where the radial pulse disappears is the palpated systolic pulse; inflate the cuff to 30 mmHg above this level
- Relax the valve gently and lower the mercury slowly and steadily at approximately 2 mmHg per second (roughly one division on the scale for each pulse sound)
- Record the systolic pressure after two beats (Phase 1 Korotkov sounds)
- Record the diastolic pressure when there is no sound (Phase 5 Korotkov sounds) for adults and when the sound becomes muffled (Phase 4 Korotkov sounds) for children and pregnant women.

If the reading needs to be repeated wait two minutes so that blood flow can be returned to normal in the arm.

Phase	Sound	mmHg pressure	
		120	Systolic
1	Sharp, clear		
		110	
2	Blowing or swishing		
		100	
3	Sharp, but softer than in 1		
		90	
4	Muffled, fading		Diastolic
		80	
5	No sound		
		70	

Fig. 9.7 The Korotkov sounds.

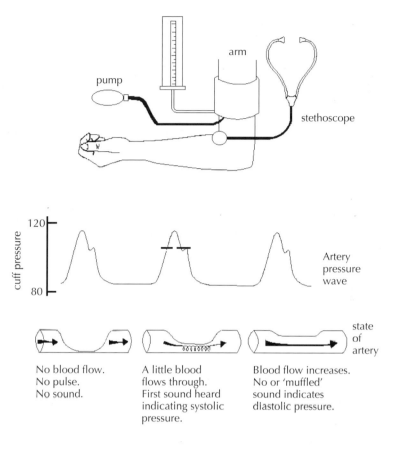

Fig. 9.8 Using a manometer to measure blood pressure.

No blood flow. No pulse. No sound.

A little blood flows through. First sound heard indicating systolic pressure.

Blood flow increases. No or 'muffled' sound indicates diastolic pressure.

🔄 Activity

Central venous pressure (CVP) is the pressure in the great veins as they enter the heart. It is measured by inserting a catheter via the arm or neck vein and moving it until it reaches the superior vena cava. The catheter is attached to a manometer containing saline or dextrose. The CVP reflects the amount of blood returning to the heart and cardiac function. Research CVP and list the advantages and disadvantages of measuring CVP. What information can be obtained from CVP measurements and what type of patient would undergo CVP measurements?

Blood pressure values

For any group of people there is no such value as a 'normal' blood pressure. There is such a thing as a 'normal' value for an individual but even this will vary through the day (Fig. 9.9) and through his/her life time (Table 9.2). It is therefore better to refer to a 'normal' range of blood pressure. The range at rest for systolic blood pressure is 100–140 mmHg (at 20 yrs) and for the diastolic blood pressure the range is 50–90 mmHg. Many factors affect blood pressure,

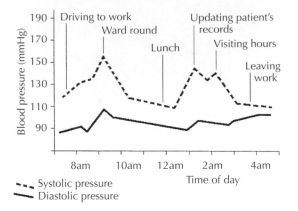

Fig. 9.9 Blood pressure variation during the day.

Table 9.2 The effect of age on blood pressure

Age Years	Blood pressure	
	Systolic	Diastolic
Newborn	80	46
10	103	70
20	120	80
60	135	89

these can include: age, gender, ethnic group, physical fitness, smoking and socioeconomic class.

A diastolic pressure which exceeds 95–100 mmHg indicates hypertension (raised blood pressure). Routine medical examinations are important since a person suffering from hypertension shows few symptoms. Hypertension imposes a strain on the heart and blood vessels which can lead to a weakening of the artery walls and consequently their rupture, or to the clogging of vessels by blood clots (thrombosis). Hypotension (low blood pressure), systolic pressure below 90 mmHg, is rarer and its most common sign is fainting. Hypotension may also result from haemorrhaging, allergic responses or response to drugs.

Resistance

Resistance is the tendency to oppose flow. Since most of the resistance occurs in the capillaries – that is in the peripheral circulation – resistance in the circulatory system is known as peripheral resistance. Resistance depends on three factors – viscosity, vessel length and vessel diameter:

Viscosity

The resistance of a fluid to flow and arises due to forces of attraction between particles in the liquid. Viscosity varies between liquids, e.g. honey is more viscous than water, blood is normally 3 to 4 times as viscous as water.

The viscosity of blood is due to the red blood cells. Some diseases, e.g. polycythaemia increase the red blood cell count and will increase viscosity; others, e.g. some types of anaemia, decrease red blood cell count and decrease the viscosity of blood.

Temperature also affects viscosity – the higher the temperature the lower the viscosity of a liquid. Shock and exposure will decrease the body's temperature thus increasing blood viscosity. Exercise on the other hand increases body temperature allowing blood to flow more easily to deliver oxygen to the tissue.

Vessel diameter

The smaller the diameter of the vessel the greater is the resistance to the movement of particles. This is due to the fact that in a narrow vessel the particles collide frequently with the walls of the vessel and lose energy – this slows down the particles and reduces the hydrostatic pressure. However, blood flow increases rapidly as the diameter of the vessel increases, flow being proportional to the fourth power of the diameter of the vessel (Fig. 9.10). Atherosclerosis is a disease that causes narrowing of blood vessels and blood flow is therefore reduced. Angina is the chest pain associated with

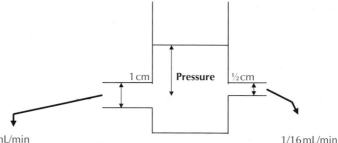

Fig. 9.10 The effect of halving
vessel diameter on flow.

If the diameter is reduced by half then the flow rate is reduced to 1/16.

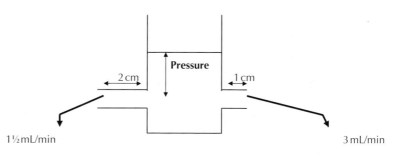

Fig. 9.11 Effect of halving length
of vessel on resistance.

Resistance to flow is proportional to the length of the vessel

atherosclerosis and occurs when the patient is exercising or under stress. This is because the reduced blood flow prevents oxygen getting to the heart muscle.

Vessel length

The longer the vessel the greater the resistance to the flow of liquid through it. There are over 60000 miles of blood vessels in the body! Increasing body mass (getting fatter) means that the body needs to increase the length of blood vessels. This increased resistance can result in hypertension (Fig. 9.11).

Flow

Blood flow is the volume of blood flowing through a vessel in a given period of time (mL/min). The lining of the vessels affects the way in which liquids flow through them. Measurements of blood flow are done by means of ultrasound making use of the Doppler effect (a shift in frequency of the ultrasound waves when they are reflected off the moving blood cells). So pressure tends to increase blood flow, whilst resistance tends to decrease flow:

$$\text{blood flow} = \frac{\text{pressure}}{\text{resistance}}$$

Two types of flow are seen.

Laminar or streamline flow

If the lining of the vessel is smooth then the fluid will flow smoothly and evenly, this is the type of flow that occurs in most blood vessels. The particles at the centre of the liquid will flow the fastest and those at the edge of the liquid will move the slowest (Fig. 9.12).

Turbulent flow

If the lining of the blood vessel is rough then flow is disorganised and has no pattern. There are more collisions and a greater loss of energy, with particles moving in every direction. Turbulent flow can be heard during the blood pressure measurement with a sphygmomanometer (Fig. 9.8). Turbulent flow also occurs when fatty plaques cause narrowing of blood vessels (atherosclerosis) or when blood vessels divide (Fig. 9.13).

So, the relationship between pressure, flow and resistance can be stated as:

blood pressure = blood flow × resistance

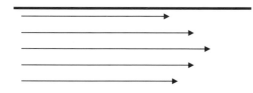

Fig. 9.12 Laminar flow.

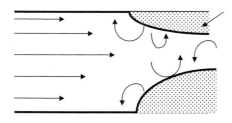

fatty plaques called **atheromas**
cause turbulent flow

Fig. 9.13 Turbulent flow.

Gases

Gases have no fixed volume or shape and occupy all the space available to them. In gases the particles are free to move about in space and continually collide with each other. The collision of the gas particles with the walls of the container results in pressure. The greater the number of collisions the greater the pressure in the container.

The physical behaviour of gases is explained in a series of laws named after the scientists who discovered them.

Boyle's law

Boyle's law states that the pressure of a fixed mass of gas is inversely proportional to its volume, when volume increases then pressure decreases, and vice versa, at a given temperature.

Pressure ∝ 1/Volume

This means that as the volume is halved the pressure is doubled, this is due to the fact that more gas particles collide with the side of the container (Fig. 9.14).

Breathing mechanism and Boyle's law

Breathing (ventilation) involves inspiration (taking air into the chest) and expiration (moving air out of the chest). Breathing movements cause a change in the volume of the thorax (chest) and therefore the pressure of the gases inside, this results in air flowing in or out of the lungs (Figs 9.15 and 9.16).

The lungs are attached to the thoracic cage by membranes called pleurae. The visceral pleura covers the outer surface of each lung and is continuous with the parietal pleura, which is attached to the inner surface of the thoracic cage. A thin layer of pleural fluid separates these two membranes. Each lung is therefore enclosed within a double-walled fluid-filled sac attached to the thorax.

Inspiration is an active process where the diaphragm contracts and flattens and the

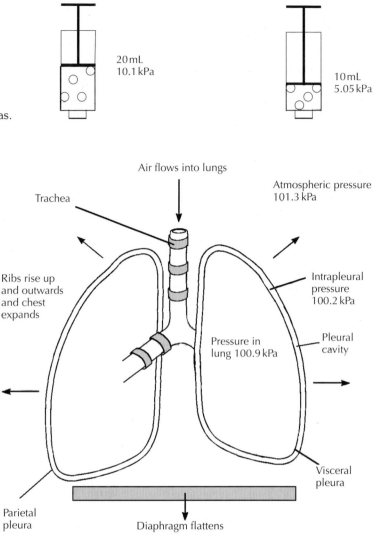

Fig. 9.14 Pressure and volume in a gas.

20 mL
10.1 kPa

10 mL
5.05 kPa

Air flows into lungs

Atmospheric pressure
101.3 kPa

Trachea

Ribs rise up
and outwards
and chest
expands

Intrapleural
pressure
100.2 kPa

Pressure in
lung 100.9 kPa

Pleural
cavity

Visceral
pleura

Parietal
pleura

Diaphragm flattens

Fig. 9.15 Inspiration (breathing in).

external intercostal muscles (muscles between the ribs) contract. The thorax increases in volume and the lung pressure decreases (Boyle's law). Since the lung volume has increased, the pressure in the lung is lower than atmospheric pressure so air rushes into lungs.

Normal expiration is a passive process where the diaphragm relaxes and moves upwards and the external intercostal muscles relax. It is the effect of gravity and the elastic recoil of the lungs that makes this process passive. The thorax decreases in volume and the lung pressure increases (Boyle's law). Since lung volume has decreased, the pressure in the lung is greater than atmospheric pressure – air moves out of the lungs. It is possible to force more air out than normal. This is an active process and is called forced expiration. This occurs during vigorous exercise or whilst playing a wind or brass instrument.

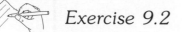

Exercise 9.2

Using the information in Figs 9.15 and 9.16 calculate the change in the intra-alveolar pressure (pressure inside the lungs) and the intrapleural pressure relative to atmospheric pressure on inspiration and expiration.

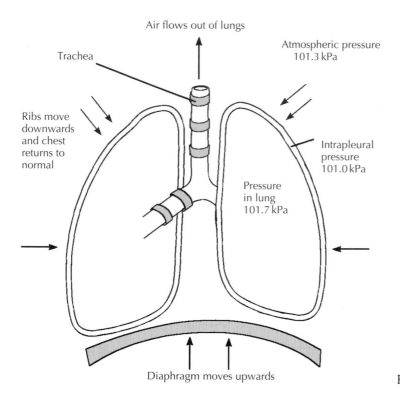

Air flows out of lungs

Trachea

Atmospheric pressure
101.3 kPa

Ribs move downwards and chest returns to normal

Intrapleural pressure
101.0 kPa

Pressure in lung
101.7 kPa

Diaphragm moves upwards

Fig. 9.16 Expiration (breathing out).

Effect of posture on breathing

Factors such as posture, obesity and pregnancy (last trimester) affect the movement of the diaphragm. When a person is supine the abdominal organs tend to be forced by gravity against the diaphragm. This makes it difficult for the diaphragm to contract and for the person to breathe. However, when a person is propped up with pillows in bed, gravity now helps to lower the diaphragm making it easier to breathe (Fig. 9.17).

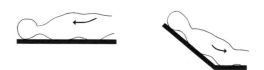

Fig. 9.17 The effect of posture on breathing.

Activity

Place yourself in the following six positions and determine which ones assist with the process of inspiration.
a)   Standing up   b)   Sitting   c)   Lying down (on a bed)
d)   Propped up with pillows, whilst lying on a bed
e)   Sitting with your knees up to your chest
f)   Bent over in half.

Chest drains

An injury, like a stab wound can cause a 'punctured lung'. A hole through the wall of the thorax and the pleural membranes allows air to move into the pleural cavity abolishing the negative intrapleural pressure. This is called a pneumothorax. When pneumothorax occurs, the lung in the affected area collapses, and movement of the chest wall no longer expands the lungs. Treatment involves releasing the air from the pleural cavity by using a chest drain (Fig. 9.18). Chest drains are known by a variety of names – intercostal drains, pleural drains and underwater seal drains.

Lung capacities

Lung capacities are measured using a spirometer. The lung capacity of a young adult male is approximately 5 litres, that of a young adult female is 4 litres (Fig. 9.19).

*   **Tidal volume** – only about 450 mL of air is breathed in and out of the lungs during normal breathing. This reflects the resis-

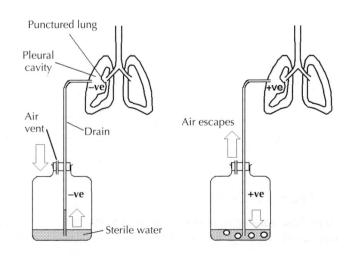

Fig. 9.18 Chest drain.

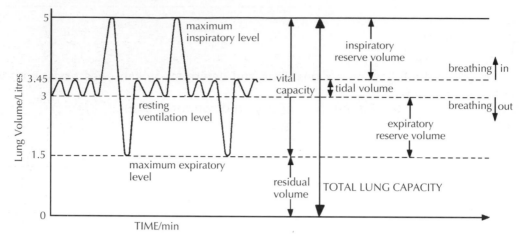

Fig. 9.19 Lung capacities.

tance of the lungs – that is how narrow the airways in the lungs are.

- **Inspiratory reserve volume** – is the extra air that can be taken in above the tidal volume, when you breathe in as deeply as possible.
- **Expiratory reserve volume** – is the extra air that can be breathed out above the tidal volume when you force air out of the lungs.
- **Vital capacity** – is the sum of the tidal volume and the inspiratory and expiratory reserve volumes.
- **Residual volume** – the air left in the lungs after the strongest possible expiration. Residual volume increases in obstructive airway diseases, since air is trapped in the lungs, however it decreases in pulmonary fibrosis, since lungs are stiff and elastic recoil is reduced.
- **Total lung capacity** – is the sum of the vital capacity and the residual volume. An increase in the total lung capacity indicates obstructive airway diseases, e.g. pneumonia or chronic bronchitis.

Peak flow meters

Peak flow meters measure in litres/minute the maximum velocity of air flow that can be produced during forced expiration. They are used by nurses for the assessment of airway functions. Low values are obtained in obstructive respiratory diseases, e.g. pneumonia. The narrower the airways the greater the resistance and the greater the pressure change needed to give air flow (Fig. 9.20).

Dalton's law of partial pressure

Dalton's law states that in a mixture of gases the pressure exerted by each gas is the same as that which it would exert if it alone occupied the space.

$$P_{total} = P_1 + P_2 + P_3 + \ldots P_n$$

P_{total} = total pressure of the mixture

$P_1, P_2 \ldots P_n$ are the partial pressures of the individual gases.

The air we breathe is a mixture of gases and contains approximately, 79% nitrogen, 21% oxygen, 0.5% water vapour, 0.03% carbon dioxide and inert gases. So for air:

$$P_{air} = P_{nitrogen} + P_{oxygen} + P_{water} + P_{carbon\ dioxide} + P_{inert\ gases}$$

The partial pressure for each gas can easily be calculated by multiplying the percentage of gas

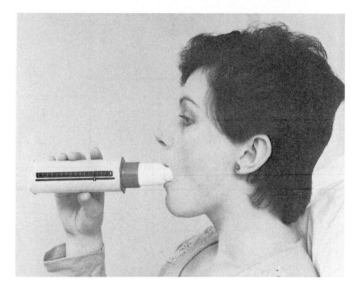

Fig. 9.20 Peak flow meter.

by the total pressure e.g. the partial pressure of oxygen is calculated as follows:

$$Po_2 = \frac{21}{100} \times 101.3 = 21.27 \, k \, Pa$$

There is a difference in the partial pressures of the gases we inspire and expire (Fig. 9.21). In the body gas exchange occurs because carbon dioxide and oxygen move in different directions due to their different partial pressures. Po_2 is high in the alveolus and so oxygen diffuses, following its own pressure gradient into the blood where the Po_2 is low. Carbon dioxide diffuses from the blood where the Pco_2 is high relative to the alveoli where the Pco_2 is low. Gases therefore diffuse independently of each other.

Henry's law

Henry's law states that the solubility of a gas, in a liquid, depends on the partial pressure of the gas and its solubility coefficient. Different gases have different solubility coefficients. The higher the solubility coefficient the more soluble the gas, e.g. carbon dioxide is roughly

Table 9.3 Solubility coefficients of gases in water at 15 °C and 1 atmosphere

Oxygen	34.1 ml O_2 per litre of water
Nitrogen	16.9 ml N_2 per litre of water
Carbon dioxide	1019.0 ml CO_2 per litre of water

23 times as soluble as oxygen in water (Table 9.3).

In blood, carbon dioxide dissolves readily and is easily transported in solution. However, oxygen is much less soluble and requires a 'carrier' for its transport. This carrier is haemoglobin. The term 'saturation' is used to describe the proportion of haemoglobin which has oxygen bound to it. Normally, arterial blood is 98–100% saturated. The amount of oxygen in blood is measured by a pulse oximeter (Fig. 9.22), which is normally placed on the patient's finger, ear lobe or toe.

As the partial pressure of a gas above a solution increases, the concentration of the gas dissolved in the solution increases proportionally (Fig. 9.23).

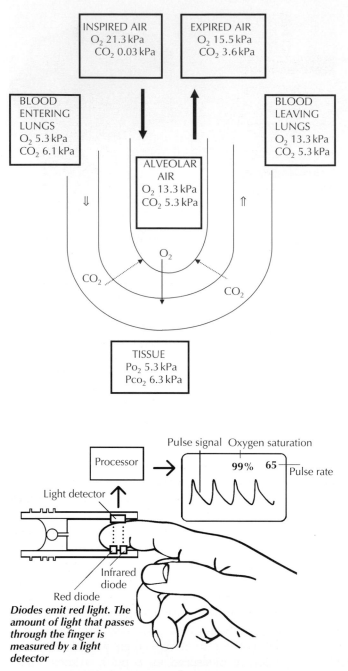

Fig. 9.21 Partial pressures of gases in inspired and expired air.

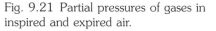

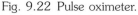

Fig. 9.22 Pulse oximeter.

At high altitudes the partial pressures of gases in the air decrease in direct proportion to the decreasing atmospheric pressure. The opposite happens below sea level, where higher than normal atmospheric pressures are experienced (Table 9.4).

At high altitudes the low partial pressure of oxygen means that less oxygen diffuses into the

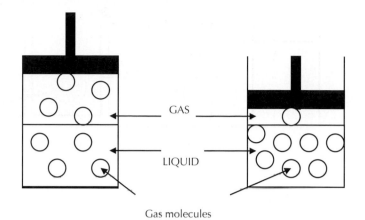

Fig. 9.23 Henry's law.   Gas molecules

Table 9.4 The effect of altitude on partial pressures

Height	Atmospheric pressure	Partial pressure of oxygen
3000 m above see level	70 kPa	15 kPa
0 m (sea level)	101.3 kPa	21.27 kPa
10 m below sea level	202 kPa	42.97 kPa

blood. This results in 'altitude or mountain sickness'. Due to the lack of oxygen people usually complain of dizziness, breathlessness (dyspnoea), nausea, vomiting and fatigue. People who live at high altitudes compensate by producing more erythrocytes (red blood cells). Newcomers can acclimatise to high altitudes over a period of time. Athletes spend weeks training at high altitudes to acclimatise before competing – as seen in the Olympic Games in Mexico City 1968.

Below sea level the partial pressure of all gases increase, which means that gases, such as nitrogen, dissolve in the blood. When a diver resurfaces too quickly, the nitrogen comes out of solution in the form of tiny gas bubbles in the tissues and blood. The symptoms of decompression sickness are paralysis, heart damage, coughing and dyspnoea ('the chokes'), and severe pains in the joints ('the bends'). Treat-ment involves recompression and slow decompression.

The Bernoulli effect

Certain types of medical equipment consist of a tube with a constriction in which the diameter gradually decreases and then increases. In such tubes the pressure is lowest at its narrowest point, often being below atmospheric pressure. This is the Bernoulli effect (Fig. 9.24). This drop in pressure can be used to entrain (draw in) a second liquid. Bernoulli's effect also applies to gases, so one gas can be entrained into another gas (e.g. Venturi oxygen mask) or a liquid can be entrained into a stream of gas (e.g. nebuliser) Figs 9.25 and 9.26.

Oxygen therapy

Oxygen is a colourless, odourless and tasteless gas. In oxygen therapy oxygen is administered in concentrations higher than those normally found in air. Oxygen therapy is used to treat

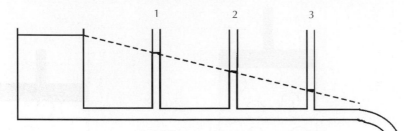

A gradual fall in pressure can be seen in all tubes

A constriction results in a large drop in pressure in tube 2,
since pressure in flowing liquids in lowest where the speed of flow is fastest

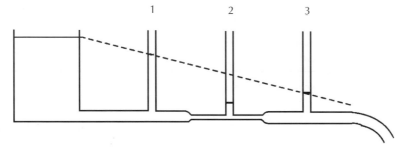

Fig. 9.24 The Bernoulli effect.

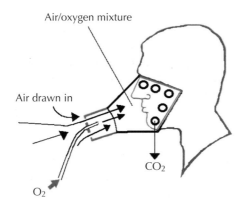

Fig. 9.25 Venturi oxygen mask.

hypoxia. Hypoxia is a condition where tissues in the body are not obtaining sufficient oxygen. There are several causes of hypoxia – anaesthesia, severe anaemia, respiratory failure,

cardiac failure, etc. and it is important that the cause of hypoxia is diagnosed before starting oxygen therapy. Oxygen may be given by face mask, nasal catheters (speculum), oxygen tents or tracheostomy tubes.

Oxygen masks

Delivery of oxygen can be fixed or variable.

- **Fixed oxygen delivery** – this is the most accurate method of delivering oxygen via a fixed performance mask, which uses a Venturi valve. It is used for any condition that requires precise oxygen delivery.
- **Variable oxygen delivery** – this is used for patients needing minimal oxygen therapy, or a variable percentage of oxygen as required by their condition. Oxygen is delivered via a nasal speculum or an oxygen mask.

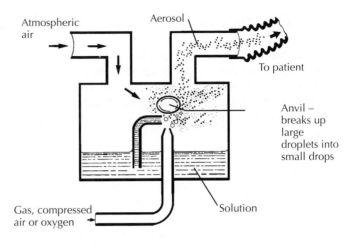

Fig. 9. 26 Gas nebuliser.

Nebulisers

In nebulisers, pressurised gas (e.g. oxygen or air) is used to form droplets of a fluid which may contain a drug (e.g. salbutamol) which is then inhaled (Fig. 9.26). Nebulisers are commonly used for patients with respiratory diseases. The gas is forced, under pressure, into the nebuliser through a narrow opening. This accelerates the gas and develops a drop in pressure inside the nebuliser (the Bernoulli effect). Due to the drop in pressure, droplets of fluid are entrained into the stream of gas, which then leaves the nebuliser and is inhaled by the patient.

Summary

- Pressure is defined as force per unit area
- There are several units of pressure; these include the pascal (Pa), millimetres of mercury (mmHg) and centimetres of water (cmH_2O)
- Pressure in a liquid acts in all directions and any change in pressure is transmitted equally to every part of the liquid
- Blood flow depends on pressure and resistance
- Arterial blood pressure can be measured using a sphygmomanometer
- Resistance to flow is directly proportional to the length of the vessel
- Flow rate is directly proportional to the 4th power of the diameter of the vessel
- Pressure of a gas is inversely proportional to its volume
- The solubility of a gas in a liquid depends on its partial pressure and solubility coefficient
- Exchange of gases in the body can be explained in terms of their partial pressures
- The Bernoulli effect states that the pressure in a liquid is lowest when the speed of flow is fastest
- Oxygen therapy is used to treat hypoxia.

▉ ▉ *Review questions*

9.1. A nurse notices on administering an enema to a patient that the solution is not flowing satisfactorily from the suspended container through the tube into the bowel. What could the nurse do to increase the flow of the enema?

9.2. Calculate the partial pressure of nitrogen in the atmosphere given that atmospheric pressure is 101.3 kPa and 79% nitrogen.

9.3. Deep sea divers use a mixture of oxygen and helium for diving instead of oxygen and nitrogen as is found in the air. Explain why they do this.

9.4. What factor determines in which direction carbon dioxide and oxygen diffuse in the lungs?

9.5. Place the following in order of increasing viscosity, giving a reason for your answer:
water, blood and plasma.

▉ ▉ *Further reading*

Jolly, A. (1991). Taking Blood. *Nursing Times*, Vol. 87 (15) p 40–43.

Blood Pressure Knowledge for Practice Professional Development Supplements. *Nursing Times* (1995). Unit 15 parts 1/3, 2/3, 3/3 Nursing Times Vol. 91, issues 14, 15 & 16.

Blood Pressure Measurement: Rational and Ritual Actions. *British Journal of Nursing*. Vol. 3 (8) pp. 393–396. D. O'Brien and M. Davidson (1994).

Pritchard, A.P. and David, J.A. (1992). *The Royal Marsden Manual of Clinical Nursing Procedures* (3rd edn). Harper & Row, London.

Hinchliff, S., Montague, S. & Watson, R. (1996). *Physiology for Nursing Practice* (2nd edn). Baillière Tindall, London.

Chapter Ten
NUTRITION AND METABOLISM

Learning objectives

By the end of this chapter the reader will be able to:
- Define the term energy
- List the various forms of energy
- Explain the theory of conservation of energy
- Give the units of energy
- Describe the role of vitamins and minerals in the body
- Describe the structure of adenosine triphosphate (ATP) and its role in the body
- Outline carbohydrate metabolism in terms of glycolysis, Krebs cycle and electron transport chain
- Briefly outline fat and protein metabolism.

Introduction

Energy is a word you use in everyday conversations. There are advertisements on TV for people to conserve energy by insulating their homes, or to drink Lucozade® or eat a Mars® bar to give them energy. Even when you are asleep you are using energy. You can feel full of energy or feel as if you need an energy boost. But what is energy and where does the body obtain it?

Definition of energy

Scientists define energy as the ability to do work. Work is defined as the force applied multiplied by the distance moved. So, if you lift any object or move a leg or arm, work has been done. If the object is too heavy to be moved then no work has been done.

Different forms of energy

Energy exists in several different forms. Energy can be divided into two broad divisions, kinetic energy and potential energy. Kinetic energy is energy of movement. Potential energy is stored energy, e.g. food contains potential energy and the body makes use of this energy when it digests the food. Kinetic and potential energy come in a variety of different forms. Some of these are:

- heat
- mechanical
- sound
- chemical
- electrical.

All of these different forms of energy are important to the body (Table 10.1).

Conservation of energy

Energy cannot be created or destroyed, it can only be changed from one form to another. The body is able to convert one form of energy to another, frequently a number of energy changes can take place (Fig. 10.1).

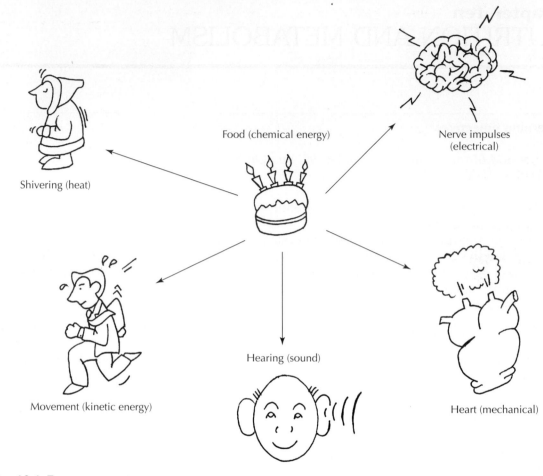

Fig. 10.1 Energy conversion.

Table 10.1 Energy in the body

Energy	Use in body
Electrical	Conduction of nerve impulses and muscle contraction
Chemical	The breakdown of chemical bonds in food and ATP
Mechanical	Pumping of the heart, churning of stomach, walking
Sound	Hearing
Heat	Maintaining body temperature, fever, shivering

Units of energy

The Système International (SI) unit for energy is the joule (J). The joule is a very small unit and so for convenience the kilojoule (kJ) is used (1 kJ = 1000 J).

The old unit of energy is the calorie (small c). The calorie is the energy required to raise 1 g of water by 1 °C. This again is a small unit and the dietary or kilocalorie is used for convenience (1 dietary calorie = 1000 calories); this Calorie has a capital C and is abbreviated to Cal. Both units are used today and Calories can be converted to kilojoules by multiplying by 4.183. The energy values of 1 g of fat, protein and carbohydrate are given in Table 10.2.

Note the high energy value for fat, approximately twice that of carbohydrates and proteins.

Table 10.2 Energy values for 1 g of substance

1 g	kJ	Cal
Protein	17	4
Carbohydrate	16	4
Fat	37	9

Exercise 10.1

Convert the following energy value from kJ/100 g to Calories/100 g
a)   apples 150 kJ/100 g
b)   digestive biscuits 2026 kJ/100 g
c)   chicken 408 kJ/100 g
Which food provides the most energy?

Bodily energy needs

The food we eat is used as a raw material for growth, repair and renewal of cells in our bodies, but its major use is for energy (Table 10.3).

The energy values of food vary enormously, those foods that have a high fat content have the greatest energy value. The way food is cooked is also important, chips contain more energy than boiled potatoes since they are fried. Butter and margarine have a similar energy value, but for health reasons it is better to eat margarine since it contains polyunsaturated fat. The energy value of food should not be confused with health value. So what is a healthy or balanced diet?

Nutrition

A nutrient is the chemical component in food that is used by the body to provide energy and to promote growth, and to repair and maintain cells. There are six classes of nutrients:

Table 10.3 Energy values of some foods

Food	Energy value (kJ/100 g)	Food	Energy value (kJ/100 g)
Chapattis	1461	Boiled potatoes	356
Bread (white)	968	Chicken	408
Skimmed milk	160	Chips	1100
Carrots	80	Cod	315
Semi-skimmed milk	206	Cottage cheese	431
Bananas	360	Lamb	804
Oranges	160	Mackerel	964
Margarine	3436	Pasta	1468
Full fat milk	320	Red Leicester cheese	1653
Butter	3376	Rice	1484

- Proteins ⎤
- Carbohydrates ⎬— macronutrients
- Fats ⎦
- Vitamins ⎤
- Minerals ⎬— micronutrients
- Water. ⎦

Each type of food provides something different and a balanced diet consists of all types of nutrients in sufficient amounts to maintain our health. For a balanced diet the following general rules should be followed:

- eat a wide variety of food
- eat mainly carbohydrates, e.g. pasta, rice and potatoes
- eat four to six portions of fruit or vegetables a day
- eat nuts, dairy products and lean meat in moderation
- use fats, salt and sugar sparingly
- drink alcohol in sensible quantities.

Vitamins

Vitamins are organic compounds. They are only needed in the diet in small amounts and are absorbed without digestion. Vitamins are used as coenzymes and antioxidants and deficiency can cause disease. There are two classes of vitamins, those that are fat soluble – vitamins A, D, E and K and those that are water soluble – vitamins C and B group. Most vitamins have to be obtained from food since they are not synthesised by the body. Heat (cooking) and sunlight can destroy vitamins. Vitamin supplements are available in all pharmacists but care should be taken since excessive intake of fat-soluble vitamins can have toxic effects, e.g. vitamin A should not be taken during pregnancy since it affects the fetus. Tables 10.4 and 10.5 summarise the source, function and effect of deficiency of vitamins.

Table 10.4 Fat-soluble vitamins

Vitamin	Food source	Function	Result of deficiency
A	Dairy products, liver, synthesised in gut from β-carotene which is found in green leaf vegetables and carrots	Needed for visual pigment, maintain epithelial cells and for teeth and bones	Dry skin, skin sores, night blindness and xerophthalmia (cornea becomes scarred and opaque), slow growth of bones and teeth
D	Fish oils, egg yolk, also synthesised in skin using ultraviolet	Helps in absorption and use of calcium and phosphorus	Failure of bones to calcify results in rickets in children or osteomalacia in adults
E (tocopherols)	Nuts, seed oils and leafy green vegetables	Inhibits red blood cell haemolysis; promotes wound healing and neural function. Prevents damage to the lipid cell membranes	Increased fragility of red blood cells, may cause anaemia
K	Liver, spinach, made by bacteria in the gut; given as an injection at birth	Synthesis of blood clotting factors	Haemorrhages due to failure of blood to clot

Table 10.5 Water soluble vitamins

Vitamin	Food source	Function	Result of deficiency
Thiamin (B$_1$)	Whole grains, yeast, pork, liver	Coenzyme in carbohydrate metabolism, needed for the production of acetylcholine (neurotransmitter)	Nerve changes, heart failure, beri-beri
Riboflavin (B$_2$)	Dairy products, meat, eggs, whole grains and cereals	Coenzyme used in carbohydrate and protein metabolism	Dermatitis, skin lesions, sensitivity to light and blurred vision, cataracts
Niacin (B$_3$) (nicotinic acid)	Meat, nuts, fish. Synthesised from the amino acid tryptophan	Coenzyme used in energy metabolism. Helps in the breakdown of cholesterol.	Pellagra (rough skin) – characterised by the 4Ds (dermatitis, diarrhoea, dementia, death)
Cyanocobalamin (B$_{12}$)	Liver, kidney, dairy products, eggs. Needs intrinsic factor from stomach for absorption	Coenzyme needed for synthesis of RNA and DNA. Growth and maturity of red blood cells	Pernicious anaemia, nervous disorders
Folic acid (folate)	Green leafy vegetables, nuts, grain products	Synthesis of nucleotides, formation of red blood cells	Megaloblastic anaemia (large immature blood cells), neural tube defects in fetus (spina bifida)
C (ascorbic acid)	Fresh fruit and vegetables	Aids tissue and wound healing. Antioxidant	Scurvy, low immune response, delayed wound healing, fragile blood vessels – petechiae (minute haemorrages), bruises

 Activity

Breakfast cereals are often fortified with extra vitamins. Look at a box of Weetabix® or cornflakes and list the vitamins you find.
Why are vitamins added to these products?

Minerals

Minerals are inorganic substances (they contain no carbon). Some are present as electrolytes, some are bound to enzymes and some act as solid structural components. The sources, function and effect of deficiency in the diet are summarised in Table 10.6.

Table 10.6 Minerals in the body

Mineral	Food source	Function	Result of deficiency
Calcium	Dairy products, green leafy vegetables, fish	Formation of bones and teeth, blood clotting, conduction of nerve impulses and muscle contraction	Loss of bone mass; rickets (children) and osteomalacia (adults) osteoporosis (over 45s, especially women)
Phosphorus	Milk, meat, fish, chicken	Formation of bones/teeth; part of RNA, DNA, ATP, kidney buffer; component of cell membrane	Deficiency is rare
Potassium	Meat, milk, whole grains	Nerve conduction and muscle contraction	Neuromuscular depression
Sodium	Salt, preserved meats and fish, processed foods	Regulates osmotic pressure of body fluids; nerve and muscle function	Dehydration, muscle cramps, kidney failure
Chloride	Widespread, found with sodium as salt	Regulates osmotic pressure and and pH of extracellular fluid; needed for gastric secretions and the transport of carbon dioxide in the blood (chloride shift reaction)	Alkalosis and muscle cramps
Magnesium	Green vegetables, beans and nuts	Part of many coenzymes; needed for normal muscle and nerve functions	Neuromuscular problems
Iron	Red meat, beans nuts, liver	Required for the formation of haemoglobin and cytochromes	Iron deficiency anaemia, fatigue, breathlessness and pallor, low immune response
Iodine	Seafood, cod liver oil, iodised table salt	Part of the thyroid hormones thyroxine T_4 and triiodothyronine T_3	Goitre (enlarged thyroid) in adults, cretinism in infants

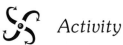 *Activity*

Iron-deficient anaemia is a common illness. The condition results in a reduction in the amount of haemoglobin or the number of red blood cells. There are many causes such as pregnancy, chronic blood loss, dietary deficiency and heavy menstruation. Find out about the signs and symptoms of iron-deficient anaemia, how it is treated and who suffers from it.

Adenosine triphosphate – ATP

Food molecules such as glucose are broken down in the body in a series of enzyme catalysed reactions. Each reaction releases a quantity of energy. Some of this energy is stored temporarily in molecules of ATP, the rest of the energy is lost as heat.

ATP is a nucleotide and consists of a molecule of adenine (organic base), the pentose sugar ribose and a chain of three inorganic phosphate groups. ATP is synthesised from adenosine diphosphate (ADP) in the cells of the body (Fig. 10.2).

The synthesis of ATP from ADP requires the addition of one phosphate group, a process called phosphorylation. This process of making bonds needs energy and is termed endergonic. When energy is needed by the body ATP is hydrolysed in the presence of the enzyme ATPase. The phosphate bond at the end of the molecule is broken and this releases a quantity of energy, this type of reaction is called exergonic. A second phosphate group can also be detached to form AMP (adenosine monophosphate) releasing a similar amount of energy (Equation 10.1).

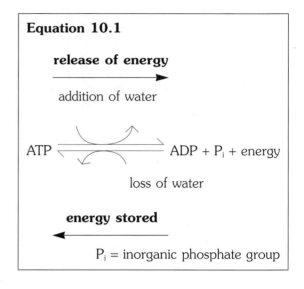

ATP is not produced and stored in large quantities. Energy is only temporarily stored as ATP and it is therefore not a store of energy as are fat and glycogen, rather a carrier of energy. ATP can be used by the cell to carry out different types of work, e.g. active transport of sodium ions (Fig. 10.3). When stores of ATP become depleted it can be re-synthesised from ADP in the cell.

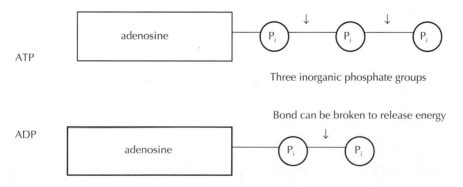

Fig. 10.2 Schematic representation of ATP and ADP.

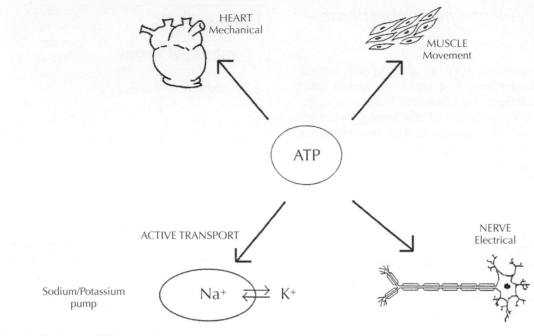

Fig. 10.3 Uses of ATP in the body.

Metabolism

Metabolism is a general term used to describe all the biochemical reactions that occur in the body to maintain life. Some of the biochemical reactions build large molecules from small molecules, i.e. are synthetic, and are called anabolic, e.g. the formation of glycogen from glucose. Anabolic reactions require energy since bonds are formed. Other reactions break down complex substances to simpler ones; such reactions are called catabolic, e.g. digestion. In catabolic reactions energy is released since bonds are broken. Some of this energy is released as heat energy and is used to keep the body warm, some of it is used to make ATP from ADP. It is important to realise that catabolic and anabolic reactions take place at the same time in the cell and it is ATP that carries the energy between these reactions (Fig. 10.4).

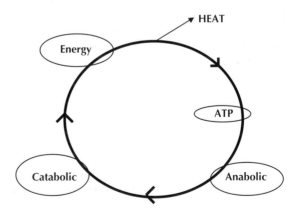

Fig. 10.4 The link between catabolic and anabolic reactions.

All the catabolic reactions that occur in the cell are collectively called cellular respiration. If cellular respiration requires oxygen then it is called aerobic respiration. If cellular respiration takes place in the absence of oxygen it is called anaerobic respiration.

Reactions of cellular respiration

A large number of the metabolic reactions in the cell involve oxidation and reduction reactions.

Oxidation

Originally oxidation was defined as either the gaining of oxygen atoms or the loss of hydrogen atoms. Today a broader definition is used, and oxidation is defined as the loss of electrons. When a substance is oxidised it loses energy due to loss of energy-rich electrons (Equation 10.2 and Table 10.7).

Reduction

Reduction reactions are the chemical opposite of oxidation reactions, that is, the gain of hydrogen atoms or the loss of oxygen atoms. Reduction reactions can also be defined as the gain of electrons. When a substance is reduced it gains energy due to the addition of energy-rich electrons (Equation 10.2 and Table 10.7).

When any substance is oxidised in a reaction another substance must be reduced so oxidation and reduction always occur together like night and day. The abbreviation **redox** is used for **ox**idation-**red**uction reactions.

Redox reactions in the body are catalysed by enzymes. Dehydrogenase removes hydrogen atoms from compounds whilst oxidase adds oxygen atoms to compounds. Most of these enzymes need coenzymes which are typically derived from one of the vitamin B group. The two most important ones are nicotinamide adenine dinucleotide (NAD+), and flavin adenine dinucleotide (FAD) – these are derived from niacin and riboflavin respectively.

Metabolic pathways

All the metabolic pathways in the body start with the digestion of proteins, fats and carbohydrates and the absorption of the breakdown products of digestion. The body then processes these nutrients through various metabolic pathways to provide the energy and the raw materials it needs.

Carbohydrate metabolism

All carbohydrates are digested to glucose. Glucose enters the cell in the presence of insulin

Table 10.7 Summary of redox reactions

Oxidation	Reduction
loss of hydrogen	gain of hydrogen
gain of oxygen	loss of oxygen
energy given out	energy taken in
loss of electrons	gain of electrons

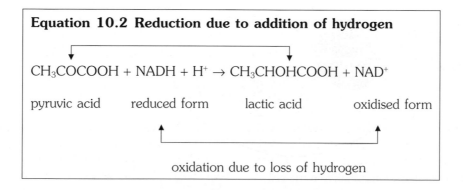

Equation 10.2 Reduction due to addition of hydrogen

$$CH_3COCOOH + NADH + H^+ \rightarrow CH_3CHOHCOOH + NAD^+$$

| pyruvic acid | reduced form | lactic acid | oxidised form |

oxidation due to loss of hydrogen

by facilitated diffusion. The complete metabolic breakdown of glucose is shown in Equation 10.3. Since the reaction requires oxygen the process is called aerobic respiration.

Equation 10.3

$$C_6H_{12}O_6 + 6O_2 \rightarrow 6H_2O + 6CO_2 + energy$$

glucose   oxygen   water   carbon   38ATP
                                       dioxide

There are four stages involved in the breakdown of glucose:

- glycolysis
- conversion of pyruvic acid to acetyl coenzyme A (acetyl CoA)
- the Krebs cycle
- the electron transport chain.

The sites of these four different stages in the cell are shown in Fig. 10.5.

Glycolysis

Glycolysis means 'sugar splitting' and occurs in the cytosol (Fig. 10.6). One glucose molecule is split into two molecules of pyruvic acid (pyruvate). (Note the acids formed in these reactions dissociate to give their anions in the body hence pyruvate is the anion of pyruvic acid, so the names are interchangeable.)

Glycolysis does not require oxygen and is an anaerobic reaction. There are three major stages.

Stage 1

Sugar activation – the glucose molecule (6C) is phosphorylated by the addition of two phosphate groups. This uses up energy, in the form of two molecules of ATP.

Stage 2

Sugar splitting – the phosphorylated glucose (6C sugar) is split into two molecules of phosphorylated 3C sugar.

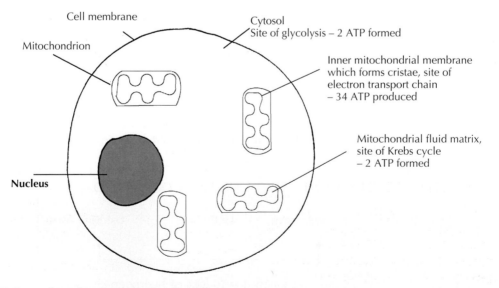

Fig. 10.5 Sites of aerobic respiration in the cell.

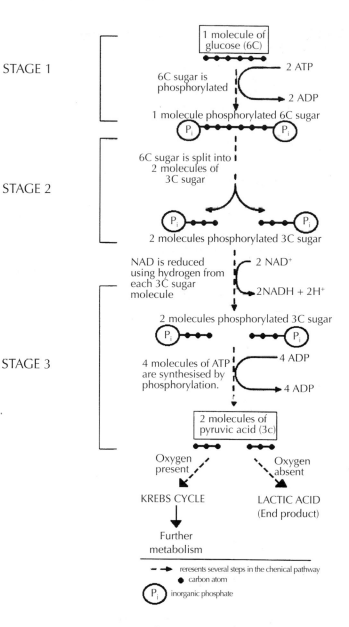

STAGE 1

STAGE 2

STAGE 3

Fig. 10.6 Summary of glycolysis.

Stage 3

Oxidation and ATP formation – the two phosphorylated 3C sugar molecules are oxidised by the removal of two hydrogen atoms from *each* of the phosphorylated 3C sugars. These hydrogen atoms are transferred to the hydrogen carrier NAD$^+$ (nicotinamide adenine dinucleotide) reducing it to NADH + H$^+$. The 3C carbon sugar is converted to pyruvic acid in a series of reactions. During these reactions a second phosphate group is added to the 3C sugar. The loss of these phosphate groups releases energy and this is used to form ATP by substrate phosphorylation (the direct transfer of a phosphate group from a metabolic intermediate to ADP).

In glycolysis one glucose molecule therefore produces:

- 2 molecules of pyruvic acids
- 2 reduced molecules of NAD$^+$
- 2 molecules of ATP

What happens to the pyruvic acid next depends on whether or not oxygen is available. If oxygen is available then the pyruvic acid will enter the Krebs cycle (aerobic respiration), if oxygen is not available it will be converted to lactic acid or ethanol (anaerobic respiration or fermentation reactions).

Conversion of pyruvic acid to acetyl CoA (aerobic respiration)

Pyruvic acid enters the fluid matrix of the mitochondria where it loses a molecule of carbon dioxide (decarboxylation) to form a two-carbon acetyl compound. If oxygen is present it reacts with coenzyme A (CoA) to form acetyl coenzyme A (acetyl CoA). At the same time two hydrogen atoms are transferred to the hydrogen acceptor NAD$^+$ forming NADH and H$^+$ (Fig. 10.7).

Anaerobic respiration (fermentation reactions)

In plants and yeasts the end product of anaerobic respiration is ethanol. However in humans and other animals the end product is lactic acid.

In anaerobic respiration there is no Krebs cycle or electron transfer chain; this means that the reduced coenzyme (NADH + H$^+$) is unable to get rid of its hydrogen atoms so it delivers them

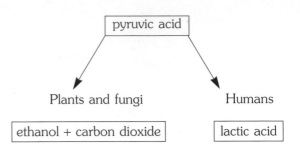

instead to the pyruvic acid. The only ATP that is generated during anaerobic respiration are the two molecules generated during glycolysis.

Aerobic respiration occurs in human muscle during vigorous exercise. The dissociation of lactic acid produces hydrogen ions which lowers the pH of the cells producing aching pain and fatigue in the muscle. Regular exercise improves blood supply, i.e. oxygen supply to the muscle, so longer periods of activity can take place.

The Krebs cycle

Sir Hans Kreb was awarded the Nobel Prize for Medicine in 1953 for his discovery of the citric acid cycle or tricarboxylic cycle (TCA). The cycle is now named in his honour (Fig. 10.8).

The main points of the Krebs cycle are:

- The starting point of the cycle is the formation of citric acid. It is formed when acetylCo A (2C) combines with oxaloacetic acid (4C)
- The citric acid goes through four redox and two decarboxylation reactions to regenerate oxaloacetic acid before the cycle is repeated

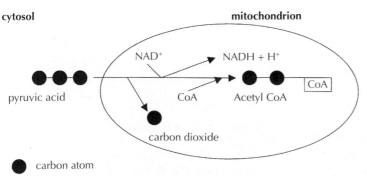

Fig. 10.7. Conversion of pyruvic acid.

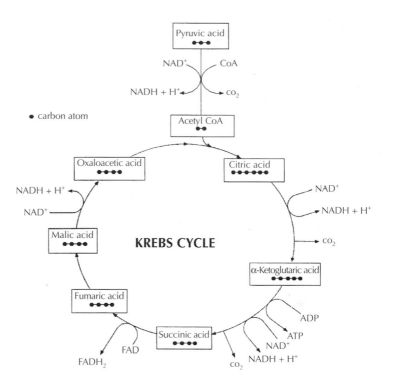

Fig. 10.8 The Krebs cycle.

- The end products of the Krebs cycle for each pyruvic acid are:

  2 molecules of carbon dioxide
  4 molecules of reduced coenzymes – $3NADH + H^+$ and $1 FADH_2$
  1 molecule of ATP

- No oxygen is needed for the Krebs cycle
- A single molecule of ATP is formed by substrate phosphorylation .

During aerobic respiration the Krebs cycle turns twice for each glucose molecule therefore 2 molecules of ATP are synthesised.

The electron transport chain

This is the final stage of aerobic respiration and it is this stage that requires oxygen. The electron transport chain is a series of reduction and oxidation (redox) reactions that occur in the inner membranes of the cristae in the mitochondria. The chain consists of a series of hydrogen and electron carriers ending with oxygen. The hydrogen atoms or electrons pass from one carrier to the next, moving downhill in energy terms. At each transfer, energy is released and used to make ATP. The final product of the chain is water.

Ten reduced $NADH + H^+$ and $2 FADH_2$ enter the chain from glycolysis and the Krebs cycle, 3 ATP molecules are produced for each $NADH + H^+$ and 2 ATP molecules for each $FADH_2$, leading to the production of 34 molecules of ATP. The formation of ATP here is called oxidative phosphorylation. Hydrogen passes from $NADH + H^+$ to $FADH_2$. When the hydrogen atom reaches coenzyme Q it breaks up into a hydrogen ion and an electron. Only the electrons continue down the chain, the hydrogen ions escaping into the watery matrix of the mitochondria.

The many electron carriers are coloured, iron containing proteins called cytochromes. Cytochromes carry only electrons. The electrons flow from carrier to carrier, each consecutive carrier having a greater affinity for the electron than the one before. This 'pulls' the

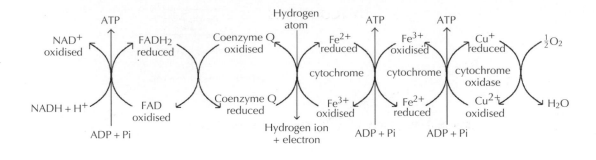

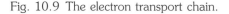

NAD$^+$　　　=　Nicotinamide dinucleotide
NADH + H$^+$　=　Reduced NAD
Pi　　　　 =　Inorganic phosphate group
FAD　　　 =　Flavin adenine dinucleotide
FADH$_2$　　 =　Reduced FAD

Fig. 10.9 The electron transport chain.

electron 'down' the cytochrome chain. The final cytochrome in the chain is cytochrome oxidase. Cytochrome oxidase is unusual in that it contains both copper and iron. It bonds with the oxygen and reduces it to an anion, O^{2-}, with the electrons received from the other cytochromes. The reduced oxygen anion (O^{2-}) then combines with the hydrogen ions to form water.

So, the final carrier in the chain is oxygen and the electron transport chain can only continue in the presence of oxygen (Fig. 10.9). The electron transport chain can be inhibited by poisons such as carbon monoxide and cyanide and certain drugs.

Carbohydrate metabolism therefore produces a total of 38 molecules of ATP:

- 2 molecules of ATP from glycolysis
- 2 molecules of ATP from the Krebs cycle
- 34 molecules of ATP from the electron transport chain.

Glycogenolysis, glycogenesis and gluconeogenesis

Glucose is used to make ATP, however excess glucose does not result in increased production of ATP. An accumulation of ATP inhibits one of the enzymes involved in phosphorylation during glycolysis and stops ATP synthesis by a negative feedback mechanism.

The liver plays a key role in maintaining blood glucose levels. When blood glucose levels increase (hyperglycaemia), glucose can be converted and stored as glycogen or fat. Glycogenesis (glycogen production) occurs principally in the muscle cells and liver. Glycogenesis lowers blood glucose levels and is stimulated by insulin secreted from the pancreas (Fig. 10.10).

Glycogenolysis (splitting of glycogen) occurs when blood glucose levels drop (hypoglycaemia). Glycogen in the liver cells is broken down under the control of epinephrine (old name, adrenaline) from the adrenal medulla and glucagon secreted from the pancreas. Glycogenolysis increases blood glucose levels (Fig. 10.10).

Gluconeogenesis occurs in the liver and is the production of 'new' glucose from sources other than carbohydrates, e.g. amino acids, lactic acid and fats. Low levels of blood glucose are particularly damaging to the brain cells since they cannot store glucose. Gluconeogenesis increases blood glucose level (Fig. 10.10).

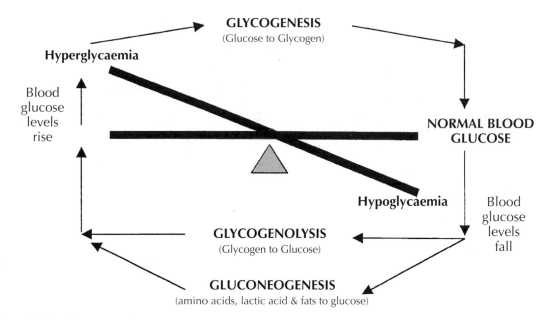

Fig. 10.10 Glucose regulation.

 ## Diabetes mellitus

A person who is unable to control their blood sugar levels within the normal range 3.5–5.5 mmol/L is termed diabetic.

There are several different types of diabetes:

Type 1 (Insulin-dependent) diabetes

Starts in childhood and results from underproduction of insulin from the β-cells in the pancreas. Treatment is by insulin injection.

Type 2 (Insulin-independent) diabetes

Starts later on in life and is connected with being overweight. About 80% of all diabetics are of this type. Insulin target cells do not respond as normal to insulin, due to some alteration in the insulin receptors. This results in a low response to insulin, a condition termed 'insulin resistance'. Treatment involves change of diet or administration of oral hypoglycaemic agents.

⚙ Activity

Nurses are expected to advise patients with diabetes mellitus on several aspects of their treatment. These include the following points:
- How and when to monitor blood sugar
- Injection sites
- Type of needles and syringes to use
- Hygiene of injection site

Find out more about these points and the role a nurse plays in the care of diabetics.

Gestational diabetes

Can develop in pregnancy and does not normally remain after giving birth. Treatment involves insulin injections or dietary change.

In diabetes glucose cannot enter the cell, blood glucose level rise and excess glucose appears in the urine (glycosuria). The presence of glucose in urine has a diuretic effect resulting in excessive urine production (polyuria), excessive thirst (polydipsia) and weakness. Diabetics are also prone to infection and wound healing takes longer due to the high blood glucose.

Lipid metabolism

Lipids are the body's most concentrated form of energy. Brain cells use glucose almost exclusively but other tissues such as cardiac muscle prefer lipids as their source of energy. The two breakdown products of lipids are glycerol and fatty acids. Glycerol is readily converted by the cells to glyceraldehyde-3-phosphate – a glycolysis intermediate. Glycerol therefore once phosphorylated can enter the glycolysis pathway where it is converted to pyruvic acid before entering the Krebs cycle. Glycerol contains 3 carbon atoms and so yields half the energy of glucose – 19 ATP.

Fatty acids undergo beta-oxidation in the liver to form acetyl CoA. This can enter the Krebs cycle directly, bypassing glycolysis. It is known as beta-oxidation as it is the carbon atom second from the acid end, in the fatty acid chain, which is oxidised. This carbon atom is referred to as the 'beta' carbon.

Beta-oxidation breaks (cleaves) two carbon atoms off at a time from the fatty acid chain. e.g.

18C fatty acid $\longrightarrow$ 16C fatty acid $\longrightarrow$

14C fatty acid $\dots \wedge\!\!\wedge\!\!\longrightarrow$ 2C acetyl CoA

The amount of energy released from beta-oxidation depends on the length of the chain of the fatty acid – stearic acid (18C) yields 146ATP, palmitic acid (16C) yields 129ATP.

Ketosis

Under normal conditions most of the acetyl CoA formed enters the Krebs cycle. However, when carbohydrate intake is restricted as in starvation or severe dieting, or when glucose is not fully utilised as in diabetes mellitus, fat metabolism is increased to compensate for the lack of glucose. The entry of acetyl CoA into the Krebs cycle depends on the availability of oxaloacetic acid, which converts acetyl CoA to citric acid. A carbohydrate deficit means that insufficient oxaloacetic acid is formed and fat oxidation is incomplete. Also the oxidation of fats for energy produces more acetyl CoA than normal. The excess acetyl CoA accumulates in the cells and is transported to the liver where it is converted to ketone bodies – acetone, acetoacetic acid and β-hydroxybutyric acid. This process is called ketogenesis. The accumulation in the body of these ketone bodies is called ketosis or ketoacidosis. Since most ketone bodies are acidic, ketosis leads to metabolic acidosis.

The signs and symptoms of ketosis are:

- deep and fast breathing – Kussmaul's respiration
- fruity smell of acetone on breath
- ketones in urine (ketonuria)
- drop in blood pH
- coma.

Protein metabolism

Amino acids are not stored in the body, however, they can be modified and used in cellular respiration. In the liver amino acids undergo deamination. An amino group ($-NH_2$) is removed from each amino acid and the carbon chain is oxidised to an acid, e.g. alanine is converted to pyruvic acid whilst aspartic acid becomes oxaloacetic acid – these can then enter the carbohydrate metabolic pathway (Fig. 10.11). The amino groups are initially converted to ammonia and then to urea, which is excreted in urine.

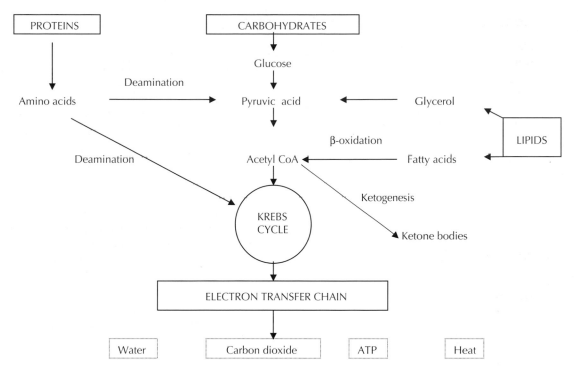

Fig. 10.11. Summary of metabolic pathways in the body.

Basal metabolic rate (BMR)

The basal metabolic rate is the energy expenditure of the body needed to maintain life, i.e. it is the energy needed to keep the heart beating, ventilate the lungs and keep the body warm. It is measured under basal conditions, which are when an individual has fasted (12–18 hrs), rested, is not stressed and is at a comfortable temperature (20 °C). Its units are kilojoules per hour.

Factors affecting BMR

- gender
- disease
- climate
- exercise
- sleep/awake.

- stress
- age
- eating
- pregnancy

Body mass index (BMI)

It is very difficult to be objective about our body mass. The press and the media are continually

Exercise 10.2

A woman weighs 60 kg and is 1.60 m tall; calculate her BMI. Comment whether she is overweight or not.

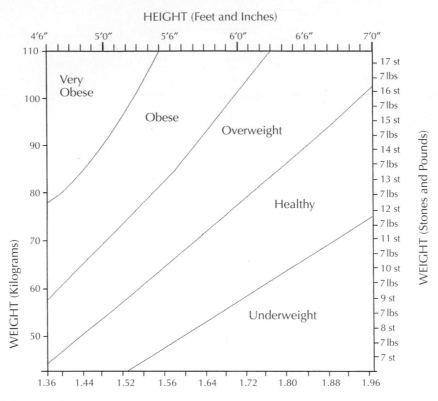

Fig. 10.12. Body mass chart.

portraying what the ideal body mass should be. However, calculating a person's body mass index gives an objective assessment of body mass.

BMI is worked out by the formula:

$$\text{body mass index} = \frac{\text{weight/mass (in kilograms)}}{(\text{height})^2 \text{ (in metres)}}$$

The ranges for BMI are as follows:

BMI	Interpretation
Below 20	underweight
20–25	ideal weight
25–30	overweight
30–40	obese
over 40	very obese

The graph in Fig. 10.12 allows you to find out your ideal body mass without doing any mathematical calculations.

As a nurse you will be able to use body mass index in various situations. A patient might be elderly and severely undernourished or suffering weight loss due to illness or treatment. Or a patient may be suffering from mental health problems such as anorexia nervosa. It will also help the nurse to explain to obese patients what their ideal weight should be.

Obesity

Obesity is common in the western world and today more people are obese than ever before. In 1991, 11.8% of men and 15% of women in Britain were obese; by 1996 the percentages had increased to 16% and 18% respectively. Obesity in children has risen even more dramatically from 5.9% (1984) to 9.5% (1994) for boys and 9.8% to 14.6% for girls.

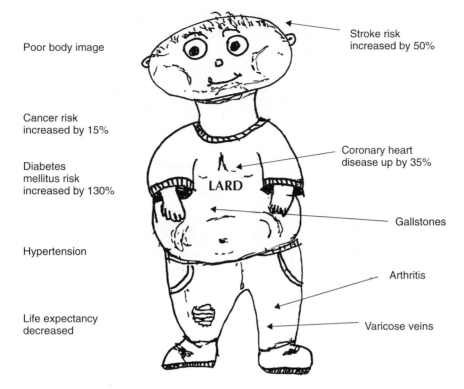

Poor body image

Cancer risk
increased by 15%

Diabetes
mellitus risk
increased by 130%

Hypertension

Life expectancy
decreased

Stroke risk
increased by 50%

Coronary heart
disease up by 35%

Gallstones

Arthritis

Varicose veins

LARD

Fig. 10.13. Health risks of being obese.

Obesity occurs when the body mass is 20% higher than the ideal. Obesity has no single cause but is a syndrome being caused by a number of factors. There are several health risks associated with being obese, these are shown in Fig. 10.13.

glycolysis, Krebs cycle and electron transport chain. 38 ATP molecules are produced
• Fats and proteins can also be metabolised to produce ATP
• Basal metabolic rate is the energy expenditure of a person under basal conditions.

Summary

- Energy is the ability to do work
- Energy comes in several different forms and these can be interconverted
- The units of energy are the joule and calorie
- Vitamins and minerals are needed to maintain a healthy body
- ATP is the biological energy carrier
- Cellular respiration can be aerobic or anaerobic
- The stages in carbohydrate metabolism are

Review questions

10.1 Why are 'starchy' foods, such as pasta and potatoes, more sustaining to the body as an energy source than 'sugary' foods, such as sweets and chocolates?

10.2 List four processes in the body that require energy from ATP.

10.3 The vitamin D content of green vegetables is not reduced by boiling, however that of vitamin C is. Explain this.

10.4 Disease, trauma and surgery can change the energy needs of a patient. Explain the energy requirements of the following patients per day.

Patient	Energy (kJ)	Protein (g)
medical patient	6300–8400	45–75
surgical patient	8400–14 700	75–125
major burns patient	14 700–21 000	125–300

10.5

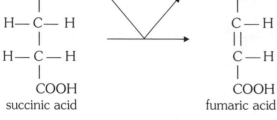

succinic acid   fumaric acid

Which of the above compounds have been oxidised and which reduced?

■ ■ *Further reading*

Sackheim, G.I. & Lehman, D.D. (1998). *Chemistry for the Health Sciences* (8th edn). Prentice Hall, London.

Hinchliff, S.M., Montague, S.E. & Watson R. (1996). *Physiology for Nursing Practice* (2nd edn). Baillière Tindall, London.

Phillips, J., Murray, P. & Kirk, P. (2001). *The Biology of Disease* (2nd edn). Blackwell Science Ltd, Oxford.

British Nutrition Foundation Homepage: http://www.nutrition.org.uk/Facts/energynut/energy.html

Chapter Eleven
ELECTROMAGNETIC RADIATION

Learning objectives

By the end of this chapter the reader will be able to:
* Explain the importance of electromagnetic radiation as a source of energy
* Describe the basic properties of waves
* Identify the existence of different types of radiation and their effects on the body (positive and negative) and describe their application in nursing practice
* Relate the hazards associated with the various forms of radiation to the health and safety precautions which are required to protect nurses
* Discuss the increasing importance of non-invasive imaging techniques in diagnosis

Introduction

Any activity that we carry out, or machine or instrument that we use requires energy. Radiation from the sun is the main source of energy in the solar system. This chapter explores the different types of radiation which comprise the 'electromagnetic spectrum' and the types of hazard that they pose to workers and patients. However, though potentially harmful, they can be used to bring great positive benefits to healthcare. This chapter also includes a section on the variety of imaging techniques that are becoming increasingly important as a diagnostic tool.

What is electromagnetic radiation?

The general term 'electromagnetic radiation' describes energy forms that are radiated from matter and transmitted in the form of waves. These waves are all of the same form but their wavelength (or frequency) determines their exact nature and properties. The types of electromagnetic waves are conveniently summarised in the electromagnetic spectrum (Fig.

11.1) and range from the highly hazardous gamma rays to long wave radio frequencies that are far less harmful.

Although most of the waves in the spectrum are not visible to the eye, the colours of the rainbow illustrate how the properties of the waves vary with changing wavelength. As you will no doubt have observed, in certain circumstances when white light travels through glass or falling rain it separates into its component colours, giving rise to a rainbow.

As Fig. 11.2 indicates, the wavelength of the radiation is the length of one complete cycle of the wave. In the electromagnetic spectrum it is measured in nanometres (nm, 10^{-9} m). The frequency of the wave is the number of waves passing through a point in one second. The unit used is hertz (Hz) or cycles per second. All electromagnetic radiation travels at the same speed of 3×10^8 metres per second. Since the speed of all electromagnetic radiation is the same, the shorter the wavelength, the higher the frequency and vice versa. This relationship is expressed in the equation:

$$\text{speed of light (c)} = \text{wavelength } (\lambda) \times \text{frequency } (\surd).$$

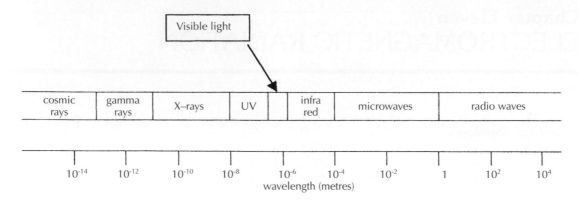

Fig. 11.1 The electromagnetic spectrum.

Exercise 11.1

The ultraviolet region of the electromagnetic spectrum is often described as consisting of three bands:

UVA: 315–400 nm
UVB: 280–315 nm
UVC: 100–280 nm

Calculate the wavelength of radiation whose frequency is measured as 1×10^{15} Hz. by using the equation above. Which band of the UV region does this radiation fall within?

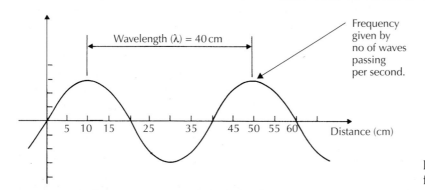

Fig. 11.2 Wavelength and frequency.

The energy in a wave is directly related to its frequency. The greater the frequency, the higher the energy of the waveform. The energy at a particular frequency is given by the equation:

$$\text{Energy (E)} = \frac{\text{Planck's constant (h)}}{} \times \text{frequency } (\sqrt{\,}).$$

The value of Planck's constant is: 6.63×10^{-34} J s^{-1}

The sun and electromagnetic radiation

The sun is the major source of electromagnetic radiation in the solar system. The energy radiated from the high temperature and high energy matter that make up the sun is necessary to support life on earth. To illustrate this,

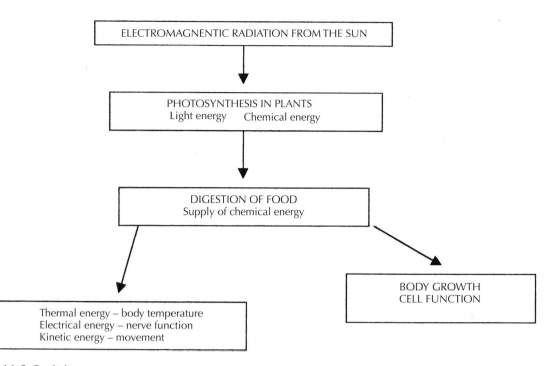

Fig. 11.3 Sunlight as an energy source.

Fig. 11.3 shows how light energy radiated from the sun is so essential for maintenance of our body functions.

Energy of radiation

It is important to be aware of the hazards that radiation can pose. Short wavelengths (high frequencies) mean that we are dealing with high-energy radiation. If the radiation is absorbed by the body this may cause unwanted and harmful chemical changes. This is particularly true with gamma and X-rays that have sufficiently high energy to ionise matter (cause the formation of ions), they are examples of ionising radiation. Conversely, radiation without this property is referred to as non-ionising radiation but under certain conditions can still be harmful through its heating effects when absorbed by the body – a concern in the current debate over mobile phone usage.

As there is a rapid decrease in the intensity (amount) of radiation with distance from its source, the negative effects of radiation can be minimised by increasing the distance between the source and the person exposed. Doubling the distance reduces the exposure to one quarter, trebling the distance reduces the exposure to one ninth and so on. This is often referred to as the inverse square law, the intensity of radiation being inversely proportional to the square of the distance.

The amount of exposure (or dose) is directly proportional to the time you are exposed to the radiation. This is not difficult to appreciate if your skin has suffered from the effects of lying in bright sunlight for too long. Shielding the skin from the radiation (by using clothing or a sun-block) is the answer to ensuring protection but still enjoying the lovely weather!

Table 11.1 Some applications of non-ionising radiation in nursing

Type of radiation	Applications	How it works
Microwaves (10^5–10^8 Hz)	Microwave diathermy	Microwaves are absorbed by water, the increase in energy raises the temperature of the water at or near the surface of the skin. The effect is rapid; care is required!
Infrared (10^{12}–10^{14} Hz)	Thermography	Diseased tissues emit larger amounts of infrared rays than healthy body tissue. Infrared detectors can be used to build up a picture of diseased tissue areas.
Visible light (10^{14} Hz)	Endoscopy	In air, light only travels in straight lines. With the use of flexible fibreoptic light pipes, light can be made to travel down parallel glass fibres linked to a tiny camera to provide an image of internal organs (as in bronchoscopy and areas of the digestive tract), otherwise invisible.
	Laser surgery	A laser beam is an intense and narrow beam of monochromatic light (a single wavelength). It can be used for cutting or destroying tissue because of its high energy concentrated on a small area as seen in keyhole surgery.
Ultraviolet (10^{15}–10^{16} Hz)	Instrument sterilisation	Germicidal lamps emit shorter wavelength ultraviolet rays (also referred to as UVC) capable of killing microorganisms and offer a useful method of instrument and equipment sterilisation.
	Phototherapy	Babies with jaundice are placed under powerful fluorescent lights that emit light at a specific wavelength that breaks down the excessive levels of bilirubin (from dead red blood cells) that cause the condition.

Activity

Investigate the information on a bottle of sunblock cream or lotion. What bands of ultra-violet (UV) radiation does it provide protection against and how do you think it achieves this aim?

Non-ionising radiation

Controlled use of the various types of non-ionising radiation has led to a number of useful treatments and techniques currently used in nursing (Table 11.1).

Radioisotopes

Radioactivity is the spontaneous emission of particles and electromagnetic radiation from the nuclei of certain unstable isotopes of the elements. Isotopes that are unstable in this way are often referred to as radioisotopes or radionuclides. For example iodine-131, the isotope of iodine with mass number 131 is radioactive, but iodine-127 is not (for more examples see Table 11.2).

The emissions from this process of radioactive decay have the ability to ionise matter that they encounter (i.e. strip electrons from atoms), hence the term ionising radiation is used to distinguish this from the other lower energy forms

Table 11.2 Examples of radioactive isotopes

Element	Stable isotope (does not decay)	Radioactive isotope
Carbon	Carbon-12	Carbon-14
Phosphorus	Phosphorus-31	Phosphorus-32
Cobalt	Cobalt-59	Cobalt-60

Table 11.3 Products of radioactive decay and their properties

Type of radiation	Nature	Charge	Atomic mass units	Range in air	Penetration
Alpha particle	Helium nucleus	+2	4	Few centimetres	Low – stopped by paper or skin
Beta particle	Electron	−1	Approx. 0	Several metres	Low – penetrates about 1 cm body tissue, can be stopped by thin metal sheet
Gamma rays	Electromagnetic radiation	nil	nil	Several hundred metres	High – reduced to low level by lead several centimetres thick, lead aprons are used to protect personnel
X-rays	Electro-magnetic radiation	nil	nil	Similar to gamma rays but less penetrating	

of radiation. The products of radioactive decay are summarised in Table 11.3.

You may be wondering how a nucleus can emit an electron, if it only consists of protons and neutrons. This can be explained by one of its neutrons emitting an electron and because of the loss of negative charge this turns into a proton:

Neutron (neutral) → Proton$^+$ + electron$^-$

Before you start worrying about the presence of radioactive carbon in the environment, it is important to remember that the quantity of radiation that is emitted by a radioisotope will be proportional to the amount of the isotope which is present (in the case of carbon-14, about 0.000 000 000 10%) and also the rate at which it decays, measured as its half-life.

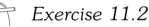 *Exercise 11.2*

Using the information above, work out the product of radioactive decay of the following radioisotopes:

i) cobalt-60 (loss of an alpha particle – alpha decay)
ii) iodine-131 (loss of a beta particle – beta decay)

Half-life

A radioisotope does not go on emitting radiation at the same rate. From the moment it is formed, its activity decays with time. The time for half of the sample to decay is described as its half-life. The rates at which different radioisotopes decay vary enormously. For example, cobalt-60 has a half-life of 5 years but carbon-14 has one of 5730 years.

Taking a 20 mg sample of cobalt-60:

- after 5 years (one half-life) 10 mg of active material will be left (half the original activity)
- after 10 years (two half-lives) 5 mg of active material will be left (one quarter of the original activity)
- after 15 years (three half-lives) 2.5 mg of active material will be left (one eighth of the original activity)

. . . and so on. In the case of cobalt-60 (and many other radioisotopes) the products of decay are themselves radioactive so the picture is often more complex Fig. 11.4.

A related measure is the biological half-life. This also measures the time for the activity of the material to be reduced by a half but in this case as a result of biological processes (elimination of body fluids). When administering radioisotopes as a part of treatment, this has to be taken into account when assessing dosage, as does the fact that the products of elimination will themselves contain radioactive materials. These will need to be handled and disposed of in such a way that workers are not at risk from significant exposure to radiation.

Radiological units and dosage

A number of different units are used to measure radioactivity. The SI unit is the becquerel (Bq) which represents one nuclear disintegration per second. Another unit is the curie, one Curie equals 3.7×10^{10} Bq. Both Becquerel and Curie were pioneers in the field of research into and use of radioactive materials.

The SI unit that relates the amount of radiation absorbed by tissue is the gray (Gy). A gray is equivalent to the absorption of one joule of energy for each kilogram of body tissue. A non-SI unit the rad (radiation absorbed dose) is also used, one rad equals 0.01 gray.

A correction factor known as the relative biological effectiveness (rbe) is used to relate the radiation damage caused by differing types of radiation to human tissue. The unit that relates specifically to the biological effect of radiation absorbed by humans is the sievert (Sv).

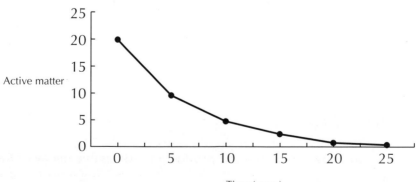

Fig. 11.4 Radioactive decay – cobalt-60.

Table 11.4 Dose–effect relationship for ionising radiation

Dose (sievert)	Effect
0.0001 (single chest x-ray)	Nil
0.001 (natural background radiation)	Nil
0.25–0.50	Decrease in white blood cell count (WBC)
0.5–1.0	Lesions, decrease in WBC
1–2	Vomiting (radiation sickness), hair loss
2–5	Haemorrhaging, ulcers, pain, death
5 or above	Fatal

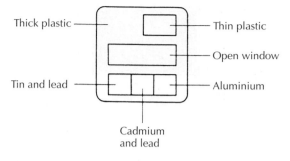

Fig. 11.5 Film badge.

1 sievert	= 1 gray × relative biological effectiveness
(Dose equivalent)	(Dose) (Quality factor)

The effects of radiation on the body will result in the damage of individual cells in the body. This may lead to cell death or cell damage. In cases of substantial doses, this damage may in turn lead to the production of damaged daughter cells and the induction of cancer (Table 11.4). If the reproductive organs are irradiated, the genetic mutations may be passed on to the children of those affected. Furthermore, irradiation during pregnancy poses the threat of fetal damage. Fortunately, ultrasound (see later) provides an alternative and safer method for fetal monitoring.

Monitoring exposure and reducing dosage

Ionising radiation cannot be seen, heard or felt – special monitors are required to detect it. To measure the exposure of radiological workers over time, the simplest method is to employ a film badge (Fig. 11.5). The film badge consists of photographic film in a plastic holder and utilises the fact that radiation exposes (blackens) photographic film. By the use of plastic and thin metal filters over the film the badge can be used to assess how much (and the type of) radiation the wearer has received.

Three important factors regarding limiting radiation exposure are time, distance and shielding:

1. **Time** – The less time spent in the radiation field the better – this can be achieved by rotating staff and careful planning.
2. **Distance** – Apply the inverse square law – the intensity of radiation received from a source decreases as the square of the distance, i.e. the level of radiation decreases rapidly as distance increases.
3. **Shielding** – The most commonly used material for shielding is lead. Lead aprons may be used for personal protection and lead screens for general shielding.

Clinical uses of radioisotopes

Diagnostic tests

Radioisotopes are used as radiotracers in diagnostic tests:

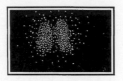

Fig. 11.6 Photo from gamma camera.

- Iodine-131   Testing thyroid function
- Chromium-51   Red blood cell analysis
- Phosphorus-32 Detection of cancer cells
                 in bone
- Iron-59   Evaluation of body iron
                 concentration

For example in testing thyroid function, the patient is fed with a small and safe dose of iodine-131. Over (or under) retention of radioactive iodine as found by urine assay indicates potential thyroid malfunction. This could be then followed by further administration of radioactive iodine, with the radiation from the incorporated iodine in the thyroid region detected by a gamma camera (Fig. 11.6).

The gamma camera detects each time a radioactive iodine atom emits gamma radiation, and it shows up on a map of the patient's thyroid. As the image fills with dots the density is higher in the regions where the thyroid cell metabolism is higher (that is, where the cells are working more actively). Areas of high emission would suggest an overactive thyroid, conversely low uptake could indicate the presence of inactive cancerous cells.

Positron emission tomography (PET)

Positron emission tomography (PET) is a non-invasive, diagnostic imaging technique for measuring the metabolic activity of cells in the human body. It is unique because it produces images of the body's basic biochemistry or function. Other imaging techniques, such as X-rays, computed tomography (CT) or magnetic

resonance imaging (MRI) – see the next section, produce images of the body's anatomy or structure which may show up abnormalities which can be related to the development of disease.

Biochemical processes are also altered with disease and may precede observable anatomical changes and may be identified by the PET technique. It is particularly useful in studying patterns of brain activity and is proving invaluable in the diagnosis of many neurological disorders such as Alzheimer's disease, Parkinson's disease, Huntington's disease, and Down's syndrome as well as the study of brain activity patterns typical of schizophrenia and depression.

A PET scan involves the use of a small amount of a particular type of radioisotope – a positron emitter. These are artificially produced by atom bombardment at very high energies in a machine called a cyclotron, have a very short half-life and emit positrons, 'positive electrons'. The positron is 'annihilated' by combining with an electron and this emission leads to the production of gamma rays (Fig. 11.7) which are detected by a gamma camera.

The positron emitter is attached or tagged to a compound that is used and metabolised by the body. Compounds similar to glucose, water, ammonia, and certain drugs may be used. The radioactive material is administered to the patient, usually by injection or inhalation and a specially designed PET scanner images how the body processes the compound or drug (Table 11.5).

Therapeutic uses

Radiation has the ability to destroy tumours. Where the radiation beam is applied externally, the most successful treatments occur on tumours that are located in areas where large doses can be given, e.g. skin or body cavities. Deep tumours within the body are much more difficult to treat, e.g. pancreas; however, implants of radioisotopes adjacent to the

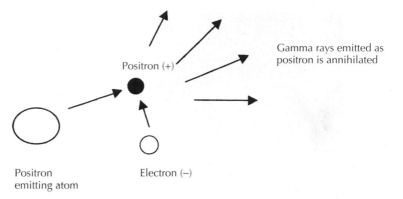

Fig. 11.7 Positron emission.

Table 11.5 PET tracers

Tracer	Radioisotope	Function
Fluorodeoxyglucose (FDG)	Fluorine-18	Following brain function
O-15 water	Oxygen-15	Measuring blood flow
C-11 carbon monoxide	Carbon-11	Cerebral blood volume
F-18 N-methylspiperone	Fluorine-18	Mapping dopamine (DOPA) and serotonin

tumour or oral administration (as in thyroid treatment) offer more flexibility.

Though radiation can have an effect on all cells, that effect is most pronounced in cells that divide rapidly. Since cancer cells come into this category, radiation has a greater effect on these than most other cells and this offers an effective and selective method of destroying tumours. Common side-effects associated with radiotherapy, e.g. hair loss and anaemia can be attributed to the fact that hair follicles and bone marrow are also types of cell which divide rapidly.

Non-invasive imaging techniques

Non-invasive techniques provide information about normal and abnormal bone and tissue structure and condition without resort to exploratory surgery or biopsy that may be time-consuming, expensive and painful. The common methods now routinely employed include X-ray methods, magnetic resonance imaging (MRI) and ultrasound.

Activity

Consider the safety implications of nursing a patient who is receiving radiotherapy. What special protocols would need to be in place if the patient were receiving an oral administration of radioactive iodine or a radioactive implant?

X-ray methods

You will no doubt be familiar with X-ray photographs (radiographs) (Fig. 11.8). These can be obtained by passing a controlled beam of X-rays through the section of the body to be examined and capturing the intensity of the transmitted rays on photographic film which is

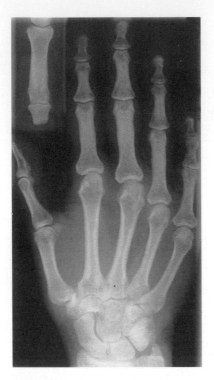

Fig. 11.8 Radiographs.

exposed on contact with the X-rays. As the degree to which the rays are transmitted depends upon the matter that they have to penetrate (bones much less than tissue), the familiar shadowy picture of the X-ray photograph is obtained.

Radiography (X-ray imaging) is the oldest and most frequently used form of medical imaging and is the fastest and easiest way to view and assess broken or cracked bones. It is also useful in detecting more advanced forms of cancer in bones but as it is a relatively crude technique, early detection of cancers requires other methods.

It is also possible to use X-rays for soft tissue investigation; higher doses are usually required to get satisfactory definition. The oesophagus (gullet), the stomach and adjacent parts of the digestive system can be more easily identified after the patient has been treated with a barium meal, the barium compound coats the lining of the stomach and makes it more clearly visible in the X-ray photograph.

Computed tomography (CT) scanning

This more sophisticated form of X-ray scanning uses the massive computing power of modern computers to interpret multiple X-ray scans to build up a two-dimensional cross-sectional picture of body tissues and organs. This is achieved by passing the patient on a horizontal bed slowly through a circular X-ray scanner (Fig. 11.9), the scanner moving around the body, taking sequences of scans recorded by detectors rather than film. Information from each of the scans is amalgamated to build up a detailed picture of the area under investigation. Each scan can be likened to a slice of a loaf of bread; when all the slices are put together the detailed picture of the whole loaf is obtained.

CT provides much more detail than traditional X-ray photographs and provides a cross-sectional view of all types of tissue, giving a detailed view of bones, soft tissue and blood vessels. It can be used to diagnose a wide range of injuries and diseases (including cancers) and

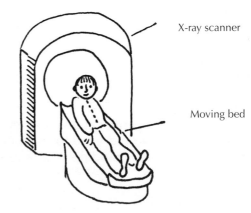

X-ray scanner

Moving bed

Fig. 11.9 Computed Tomography.

to guide radiation treatment for tumours and investigative biopsies. In investigating certain tissues or blood vessels a contrast agent (of different opacity and generally containing iodine compounds) to enhance the visibility of the tissue may have to be used.

Although CT involves exposing the patient to multiple scans, more sensitive detection methods mean that much lower doses can be used. The typical radiation dose from a CT scan is equivalent to the amount of natural background radiation received over a year. As with all X-ray examinations, to ensure maximum safety of the patient the abdomen and pelvis are shielded with a lead apron except where this is the area that is being imaged.

Magnetic resonance imaging (MRI)

Although the flat bed scanner used for MRI (magnetic resonance imaging) looks similar to that used for CT, this is a completely different imaging method because it irradiates the patient with radio frequency waves in the presence of a strong magnetic field. It does not rely on ionising radiation at all.

The magnetic field is used to line up the nuclei of atoms (they behave like small magnets). Radio waves are tuned to interact with specific nuclei (most commonly protons, the nuclei of hydrogen atoms) in this magnetic field. The nuclei are first 'excited' and then allowed to 'relax' thus emitting radio signals. These provide the information which can be computer-processed to form an image mapping the abundance of material containing hydrogen atoms. With proton-based MRI, as water is the most abundant hydrogen containing material in the body, an MR image will be able to detect differences in the water content and distribution in body tissues. In this way even the grey and white matter of the brain can easily be distinguished. A MRI examination consists of a number of imaging sequences, each lasting a

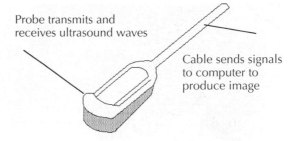

Probe transmits and receives ultrasound waves

Cable sends signals to computer to produce image

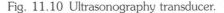

Fig. 11.10 Ultrasonography transducer.

few seconds to 15 minutes, the whole process may last up to an hour.

Ultrasound (ultrasonography)

Ultrasound imaging obtains images from inside the human body through the use of high frequency sound waves in a manner similar to the sonar used by bats and by ships at sea. The sound waves emitted bounce against internal organs and the echoing waves which return can be used to identify the distance of the object, its size and uniformity. The waves are able to 'find' the boundary between different types of tissue, e.g. muscle and bone. An ultrasound 'transducer' is used which provides both a loudspeaker (to emit the sounds) and a microphone to receive them (Fig. 11.10). These recorded waves are processed and displayed by a computer creating a 'live' real-time picture on the monitor which can be captured on videotape or displayed as a series of still images.

A particular benefit in obstetric ultrasound (the use of sound waves to visualise and determine the condition of a pregnant woman and her embryo or fetus) is that the technique does not use X-rays to produce an image (Fig. 11.11). Neither the mother nor her unborn child is exposed to ionising radiation.

Doppler ultrasonography is an application of diagnostic ultrasound that can detect the direc-

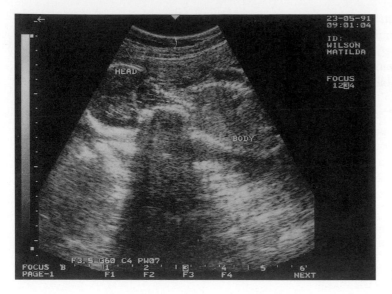

Fig. 11.11 Ultrasound scan.

Table 11.6 Some applications of imaging techniques

	Traditional radiography (X-rays)	Computed tomography (CT)	Magnetic resonance imaging (MRI)	Ultrasound
Cardiovascular system (heart, blood vessels)	None	Detection of vascular diseases	Coronary artery disease, heart problems	Evaluation of arterial blockages and blood flow
Central nervous system (brain, spine)	None	Head injuries, brain tumours and diseases	Brain tumours, strokes, multiple sclerosis, brain abnormalities, pituitary gland	None
Digestive, urinary & respiratory systems	Chest radiography, urinary tract investigation, lower GI tract	Cancer diagnosis, injury to internal organs	None	Abdominal imaging
Musculoskeletal system	Fracture identification, arthritis in bones (diagnostic)	Spinal and skeletal injuries, osteoporosis	Sports related injuries, joint disorders	Tendon tears, fluid collection in muscles
Reproductive system & mammography	Mammograms	None	Reproductive system examination	Fetal imaging, guiding needle biopsies, breast imaging

tion and speed of movement by measuring changes in frequency of the echoes reflected from moving structures (the Doppler effect is also used by the police to measure the speed of moving vehicles). It is now an important method used to evaluate blood vessels and blood flow, providing the opportunity for real-time imaging that assists in monitoring the functioning of the major arteries and veins of the body and the heart. It is also used to check the blood flow to the placenta in fetal monitoring.

Choice of imaging techniques

The technique of choice for non-invasive imaging will depend both on the clarity and nature of the information provided by the image formed and also safety considerations. Both X-ray methods and MR imaging are avoided in pregnancy but otherwise they are considered safe as long as appropriate precautions are taken. Ultrasound has been used in fetal monitoring for over 30 years and there is no evidence of damage to fetus or mother. The applicability of these methods is summarised in Table 11.6.

Summary

- The electromagnetic spectrum describes the different types of energy that are transmitted in the form of waves, ranging from gamma rays to radiowaves
- The sun is a major source of electromagnetic radiation
- The energy of a waveform is directly proportional to its frequency
- We distinguish between ionising radiation and non-ionising radiation in terms of the effect the radiation has on matter
- Radioisotopes are atoms with unstable

nuclei that emit particles and ionising radiation as they decay
- The half-life of a radioisotope is the time taken for 50% of the sample to decay
- Ionising radiation is useful in its ability to kill cancerous cells
- Ionising radiation is used in a variety of diagnostic and imaging techniques – e.g. X-ray, CT and PET scans
- Imaging techniques that do not use ionising radiation are MRI and ultrasound
- Control of dosage (time, distance shielding) is essential in minimising the harmful effects of ionising radiation on patients and workers.

Review questions

11.1.   What type of radioactive decay do you think is occurring in the following examples?
i)   radium-226 → radon-222?
ii)   sodium-24 → magnesium 24?

11.2.   Radioactive phosphorus has a half-life of approximately 14 days. How long would it take for the activity of this sample to reduce to one eighth of its original amount?

11.3.   Positron emission tomography (PET) and computed tomography (CT) both use radiation to provide images of the body (or parts of it) to assist in diagnosis and yet the two scanning techniques are very different. Why?

11.4.   Patients often have metal objects in their clothing and also possibly implanted in their bodies. How might the presence of such objects affect the performing of a CT or MRI scan?

11.5.   When on a sunbed or having phototherapy, what protective equipment should you wear?

■ ■ *Further reading*

Hickman, R. & Caon, M. (1995). *Nursing Science: Matter and Energy in the Human Body* (2nd edn). Macmillan, Melbourne.

Cree, L. & Rischmiller, S. (1995). *Science in Nursing* (3rd edn). Baillière Tindall, London.

Medical Imaging Techniques. Homepage at: http://cfi.lbl.gov/~medhome.html

Medical Graphics and Imaging Group. University College London and UCL Hospitals. Homepage: http://www.medphys.ucl.ac.uk/mgi/

Chapter Twelve
TEMPERATURE AND HEAT

Learning objectives

By the end of the chapter the reader will be able to:
- Differentiate between heat and temperature
- Give the units of temperature
- Describe the theory behind temperature measurement
- Discuss the importance of temperature measurement as a diagnostic test
- Describe the ways in which bodies gain and lose heat and how unwanted changes may be controlled.

Introduction

Taking a patient's temperature is one of the most straightforward tasks for a nurse; its frequency indicates the importance of the relationship between maintaining correct body temperature and homeostasis. Consequently, understanding ways that temperature control may be achieved (both internally and externally) are important in understanding the treatment and avoidance of many medical conditions.

Heat and temperature

Heat is a form of energy. We are all familiar with the fact that heat energy is produced when fuels burn, electricity is passed through conducting wires or food is digested in our bodies but what exactly is heat energy? All matter contains heat energy and this is because of the movement or vibrations of the particles (atoms, molecules or ions) that make up the material under consideration. The particles that make up matter are all vibrating to a greater or lesser extent. An increase in heat energy is associated with increasing vibrations in the material, a reduction of heat energy means that the extent of these vibrations has been reduced.

Temperature is a measure of the 'relative degree of hotness or coldness' of a body, related to the freezing and boiling points of water, which are fixed as simple numerical figures (Fig. 12.1). Temperature is not a measure of the amount of heat energy contained in a body. That will depend on the size of the body (a cup of water will contain far less energy than a bath full of water at the same temperature) and also the nature of the material itself.

Substances require differing amounts of heat energy to raise their temperature by the same amount. This is indicated by the specific heat capacity of the material in question, the amount of energy to raise 1 kg of the material by 1 °C. The value for water is 4.2 kJ but for mercury it is only 0.14 kJ.

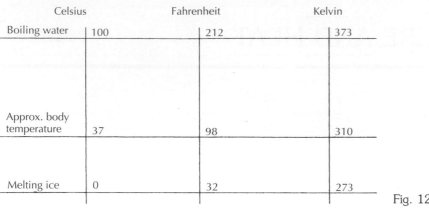

	Celsius	Fahrenheit	Kelvin
Boiling water	100	212	373
Approx. body temperature	37	98	310
Melting ice	0	32	273

Fig. 12.1 Temperature scales.

Exercise 12.1

How much heat energy is required to raise the temperature of 70 kg of water by 2 °C? This value has some significance if you consider 70 kg to be an average body weight and the human body to be made up substantially of water. A 30 g bar of chocolate has an energy value of about 600 kJ by the way!

Temperature scales

The most commonly used temperature scale and the one used in clinical practice is the Celsius (or centigrade) scale. The Celsius scale is divided into 100 degrees between 0 °C, the lower fixed point (the melting temperature of ice) and 100 °C, the upper fixed point (the boiling point of water). It should be added that these fixed points are determined at normal atmospheric pressure, as the values are dependent on the air pressure when the measurement is taken.

Two other temperature scales should be mentioned. The SI unit of temperature is the kelvin (K). It employs the same divisions as the Celsius scale but recognises that the absolute zero of temperature will correspond to the situation where all molecular motion has completely ceased. This situation (0 K) cannot actually be obtained but were it to exist the tempera-ture would be −273 °C! Hence 0 °C is equal to 273 K and so on.

Although the Fahrenheit (F) scale is no longer officially used in the United Kingdom, it is still used elsewhere and many older people grew up when it was universally used. For this reason it may be useful to be able to convert temperatures to and from this scale in which the freezing point of ice is 32 ° and the boiling point of water 212 °F. This is easily done using the simple formula:

Exercise 12.2

Using: $°C = 5/9 \times (°F - 32)$ and $°F = \left(\frac{9}{5}°C\right) + 32$
(a) Convert 37 °C to Fahrenheit
(b) Convert 68 °F to Celsius
(c) Express 100 °C in degrees kelvin

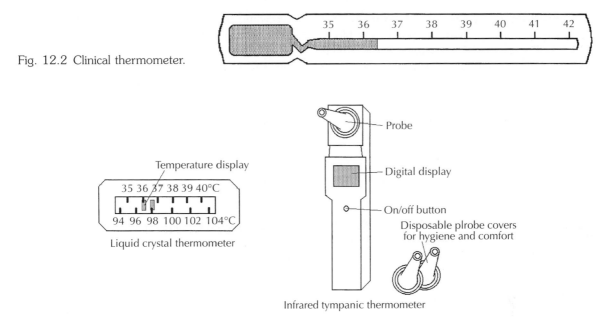

Fig. 12.2 Clinical thermometer.

Liquid crystal thermometer

Infrared tympanic thermometer

Fig. 12.3 Typical non-mercury thermometers.

$$°C = \left(\frac{5}{9}\,°F\right) - 32$$

$$°F = \left(\frac{9}{5}\,°C\right) + 32$$

Measurement of body temperature

Devices for detecting changes in temperature rely on measuring the change in physical property of a substance or material as its temperature changes. The most common way this is done is by using the way a liquid, usually mercury, expands as it warms up (and contracts as it cools down). This occurs relatively rapidly as mercury has a lower specific heat capacity than many other liquids. This type of thermometer consists of a glass bulb (reservoir) attached to a tube which measures the expansion or contraction of the liquid as it is heated or cooled. Fig. 12.2 illustrates the clinical thermometer; the narrow constriction between bulb and tube ensures that the column

of mercury does not fall immediately the temperature has been taken. Indeed, it has to be shaken down before another reading can be taken.

A drawback with the mercury thermometer is the spillage of the toxic mercury if the device is broken. This has led to the more frequent use of less hazardous and disposable thermometers (Fig. 12.3). Other temperature measuring devices important in clinical practice are summarised in Table 12.1.

In taking body temperatures, it is important to realise that though the normal body temperature is generally accepted to be 36–37°C, significant variations from this figure do occur in normal conditions. Firstly we must distinguish between core and peripheral (surface) body temperatures as the typical values below illustrate:

Core (internal) temperature	37°C
Axilla (armpit) temperature	36.5°C
Surface temperature – scalp	35°C
Surface temperature – foot	29°C

The lowest temperatures are to be found at the body's extremities – at these points the blood which is the carrier of heat around the body has already given up much of its heat energy – on

returning to the core it will be re-heated prior to its next journey round the body.

The activity level of the body immediately prior to the measurement being taken must be

---

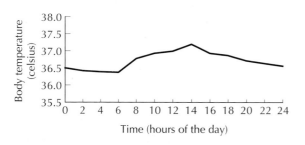

Exercise 12.3

The rise in temperature following ovulation is very small. What precautions do you think would need to be taken to ensure that an accurate temperature is recorded?

---

considered and thirdly, so must the time of day (Fig. 12.4). Another variation in core temperature occurs during the menstrual cycle. Progesterone released following ovulation causes a small temperature rise of about 0.5°C. As the progesterone level falls, so does the temperature. This can be used to map the progress of the cycle if natural birth control is being practised or if pregnancy is wanted.

Latent heat

You should recall the interconversion of the three states of matter:

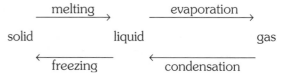

Remember the types of structure associated with these three states:

- Solid – particles tightly held in a rigid structure by forces between the particles
- Liquid – particles free to move but still held together
- Gas – individual particles with no forces holding them together.

Progressive addition of heat energy is required for the material to heat up (the parti-

Fig. 12.4 Daily body temperature fluctuations.

Table 12.1 Temperature measuring devices

	How it works	Typical application
Thermistor	Change in resistance of semi-conductor (current flow is measured)	Rectal probe (continuous monitoring)
Liquid crystal thermometer	Change in colour of liquid crystal with temperature is observed	Surface skin temperature
Infrared tympanic membrane thermometer	Intensity of infrared radiation emitted by tympanic membrane (ear drum) is measured	Instant, accurate measurement of core body temperature

cles to vibrate faster) and eventually change state. When the substance changes state additional energy is required for the particles to break out of the rigid structure (solid to liquid) or free from the liquid (liquid to gas). This is neatly illustrated by following the temperature rise of the solid naphthalene (used in mothballs) as it is steadily heated through its melting point. What we see is that when the melting point is reached, even though further heat is applied, the temperature does not increase until the material has melted; extra energy is required to reorganise the material as a liquid. This additional heat energy is called latent heat and is the energy taken in or given out when a material changes its state. In the changes resulting from cooling, (condensation and freezing) heat energy is given out rather than taken in as the change occurs.

Comparing the latent heat value for water with its specific heat capacity value shows that a substantial amount of energy is required for these changes of state:

- specific heat capacity $4.2\,kJ\,kg^{-1}$
- latent heat of fusion
  (ice to water) $336\,kJ\,kg^{-1}$
- latent heat of vaporisation
  (water to steam) $2260\,kJ\,kg^{-1}$.

This accounts for the very severe heating effects of scalding when steam condenses on human flesh – due to both the temperature of the hot water vapour and the latent heat emitted as the steam condenses on the surface!

Regulation of body temperature by evaporation

Latent heat is important in understanding one of the main mechanisms the body can use to reduce its temperature and keep within safe operating limits. In order for water or sweat on the surface of the skin to evaporate, additional heat energy has to be drawn from the body for this to occur (latent heat is required, as explained above). This provides a constant cooling effect of the body and one that can be regulated on demand by changes in the rate of sweat production. It is estimated that this accounts for about 20% of total heat loss by the body in normal conditions over the course of a day. Dampening the skin with water, which will then evaporate, can enhance this cooling effect. The rate of evaporation will be faster if there is significant air movement to blow away the evaporated water. Conversely, in very humid conditions, where there is already a high content of water vapour in the atmosphere, the rate of evaporation will be slowed down as the air becomes saturated with evaporated water.

Transmission of heat

There are three ways heat is moved or transferred: conduction, convection and radiation. All three are important in terms of understanding how heat loss from the body occurs and how it can be controlled.

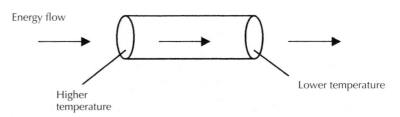

Energy flow

Higher temperature

Lower temperature

Fig. 12.5 Conduction of heat.

Conduction

Conduction is the transfer of heat in solids, liquids and gases (or from one substance in contact with another). It is due to the molecules colliding with each other and transferring their heat energy through the material. (Fig. 12.5).

Heat energy will move from a warmer area to a colder area by this process. This heat transfer occurs rapidly in metals which are good conductors of heat. Most materials other than metals are not good conductors and they are referred to as heat insulators. This is easily appreciated if you compare picking up a hot saucepan with a metal handle rather than one with a wooden or plastic handle. The wood or plastic does not conduct the heat from the rest of the saucepan, it insulates you from the heat.

The measure of the efficiency of a particular material in the transfer of heat is called its thermal conductivity. Metals have high thermal conductivity values and they feel cold to the touch as the rapid conduction of heat away from the hand is sensed through the skin.

Though heat loss by conduction from human bodies is relatively limited, its prevention by surrounding the body with insulating materials is significant. Air is an excellent insulator – loose clothing and bedding which provide a layer of air around the patient will reduce heat loss significantly.

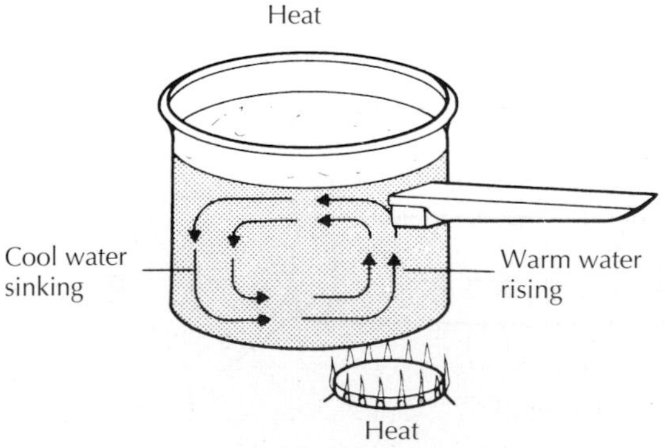

Convection

This is the transfer of heat where the heat travel is due to the actual movement of a fluid (a liquid or a gas). This movement occurs when a fluid heats up, it becomes less dense, rises and produces what is called a convection current as it is replaced by colder fluid (Fig. 12.6). This effect can be observed when the water in an electric kettle or saucepan is heated and the movement of the water can be seen.

If a mobile is placed above a fire or radiator, the movement of the mobile demonstrates the air turbulence caused by the convection current of warmer air. Some heat loss from the body occurs by convection as the body will generally be somewhat warmer than its surroundings.

Radiation

Hot bodies, in particular those above 100°C, emit rays (infrared rays) which on impact with other bodies are absorbed, causing a rise in temperature. (Fig. 12.7). The most significant

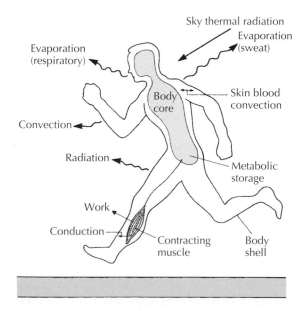

Fig. 12.6 Convection currents in a heated liquid.

Heat

Cool water sinking

Warm water rising

Heat

Fig. 12.7 Heat production during exercise.

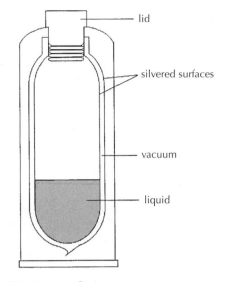

lid

silvered surfaces

vacuum

liquid

Fig. 12.8 Vacuum flask.

example of this is the heating effect of the rays emitted from the sun. You will also have noticed the effect of radiant heat sitting close to a hot fire. Being less than a temperature of 100°C, human bodies do not radiate a large amount of heat. However, different types of surface absorb radiation by differing amounts, dark surface much more than light or white ones. Radiation also tends to be reflected from shiny, polished surfaces.

The vacuum flask

The vacuum flask (Fig. 12.8) is an excellent illustration of how transmission of heat can be minimised and a liquid stored in the flask can be kept at a constant temperature for a long period of time. This allows the storage of both hot and cool liquids with minimal change in temperature. Though we may be more familiar with using a vacuum flask to keep our coffee or tea hot, it is frequently used to keep liquefied gases (e.g. liquid nitrogen) at very low temperatures. In such circumstances it is usually referred to as a Dewar flask, after its inventor, Sir James Dewar.

Temperature homeostasis – heat balance in the body

It has been estimated that if the body had no means of losing heat, its temperature would rise by about 1 °C each hour. The heat in the body is generated by cell metabolism, converting the chemical energy of digested food into other forms of energy, substantially heat energy. As this metabolic process is continuous, though not constant, the body must also lose heat energy at such a rate that there is not a build up of heat and a corresponding increase in temperature. Overall, the heat gain from metabolism and other sources must equal the heat losses from the surface of the body. This is the essence of temperature homeostasis.

The hypothalamus – the body's thermostat

The body's thermostat is the hypothalamus, monitoring the temperature of blood being pumped through the brain; further information is provided by the skin's temperature receptors. There are a number of ways in which the body can increase temperature on demand including:

- metabolic stimulation, increasing heat production
- vasoconstriction (narrowing) of blood vessels within the skin, reducing heat loss through the skin
- shivering – contractions of skeletal muscles producing heat energy.

Conversely, heat losses will occur via the following ways:

- convection (also some radiation and conduction) of heat particularly from exposed and uninsulated skin surfaces
- vasodilation (expansion) of blood vessels within the skin, increasing heat loss through the skin

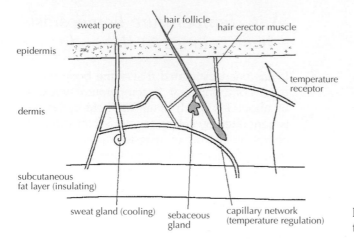

Fig. 12.9 The structure and function of the skin.

- increased evaporation of sweat from skin
- exhalation of hot air from lungs
- elimination of faeces and urine.

In addition, behavioural changes by the individual will be important too, responding to the signals of feeling hot or cold in an appropriate way. For example, the ingestion of hot food and drink and seeking warm surroundings will contribute to heat gains if the requirement is recognised and able to be acted upon.

The role of the skin in heat regulation

The skin (Fig. 12.9) is the interface between the internal tissues of the body and the surrounding environment. It is at the skin that evaporation of sweat and heat losses occur. If there are substantial layers of insulating fat beneath the dermis, these heat losses will tend to be reduced. The skin also contains temperature receptors that feed information back to the hypothalamus about 'the temperature outside'. The networks of blood capillaries in the dermis also have an important function in temperature control. Vasoconstriction (narrowing) or vasodilation (expansion) of these blood vessels can vary the rate of blood flow at the skin by a factor of as much as 100%. This is achieved by the constriction or dilation of connecting blood vessels which divert blood flow to or away from the capillary networks as it is required (Fig. 12.10). For body cooling the flow of blood is increased to enable heat loss at the skin's surface; conversely if body heat needs to be retained, the flow is reduced.

Fever

Fever or pyrexia should be mentioned here. Fever results from the resetting of the hypothalamus 'thermostat' to a higher temperature. The body can be considered to be running at a higher temperature and not necessarily out of control. The onset of fever corresponds to the body's response to the resetting of the core temperature value and does not indicate that the regulatory system is not working. There are many possible causes of a fever but it is most commonly the result of infection. It is argued that in these circumstances the fever is in many ways beneficial, as the body's immune response is more effective at higher temperatures. Drugs used to control fever, such as aspirin and paracetamol, are called antipyretics.

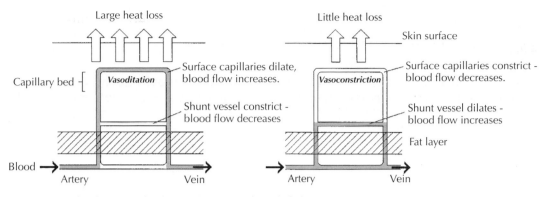

The shunt vessel (arteriovenous or AV shunt) links/bypasses
arteriole and venous blood supply to the capillary network.

Fig. 12.10 Vasoconstriction and vasodilation of skin capillaries.

Control of abnormal body temperatures – hypothermia and hyperthermia

There are a number of circumstances where the normal temperature regulatory mechanisms are no longer effective. These include:

- Malfunction of the hypothalamus due to cerebral trauma – head injuries, brain surgery, cerebrovascular accidents
- Effects of toxic substances, in particular, some bacterial or viral infections
- Dehydration – with corresponding loss of sweating function
- Prolonged exposure to extreme temperatures (hot or cold).

Hypothermia

This condition is most likely to result from an injury in a cold environment, submersion in cold water, or a prolonged exposure to low temperatures without adequate protective clothing. It may also be deliberately induced, reducing core body temperature to 30 to 32 °C, prior to cardiac or neurological surgery. The greatest susceptibility is amongst infants and the elderly. Infants have a larger body surface relative to total mass than adults, allowing more rapid heat loss. The elderly have a lower metabolic rate than the young so it is more difficult for them to maintain normal body temperature when the temperature of the surroundings is low. Ageing is also accompanied by a reduction in the ability to detect temperature changes and take appropriate action. Note also that immersion in cold water can cool the core body temperature much more rapidly than exposure to cold air, because the thermal conductivity of water is 32 times greater than that of air. Severe hypothermia (body temperature below 30 °C) is associated with marked depression of cerebral blood flow and oxygen requirement, reduced cardiac output, and decreased arterial pressure.

Active core re-warming techniques are required in severe hypothermic victims but must be administered with great care due to the possible life-threatening conditions that arise during stabilisation and resuscitation. Techniques employed include the administration of preheated intravenous fluids and warm, humidified air or oxygen (heated to 42 to 46 °C). Passive rewarming methods, suitable for mildly hypothermic victims and as supplementary treatment in cases of more severe hypothermia, include heat packs to arms and groin areas, heating lamps, warmed blankets, and warm air heated 'sleeping' bag devices.

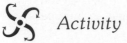

Activity

Hypothermia is an avoidable condition. What precautions would need to be in place to ensure it did not occur in an elderly person living alone in a relatively cold climate?

Hyperthermia

The onset of hyperthermia is associated with situations where heat gain in the body (from internal or external sources) is not being offset by corresponding heat losses to the environment. There is then the danger that core body temperature will rise to levels at which there is a complete breakdown in the body's temperature regulatory mechanism and without intervention, death can result. Though mostly associated with overexposure to hot environments, the condition can also occasionally be triggered in susceptible patients by exposure to some anaesthetics (malignant hyperthermia or hyperpyrexia). As with hypothermia, there is a greater predisposition to this condition in the elderly.

Treatment requires immediate cooling. Cooling by promoting evaporation (misting the body with water or washing the body with tepid water) and encouraging heat loss by the conventional methods of conduction, convection and radiation are all important. With excessive fluid loss from sweating, rehydration will also need to be considered. Airway management may be required – aspiration and seizures are common in these circumstances.

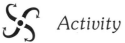

Activity

Find out what other methods of cooling are used for patients with hyperthermia and work out whether they involve conduction, convection or radiation as the means of increasing heat losses.

Summary

- Heat is a form of energy, temperature is the measure of the relative degree of hotness of a body
- Temperature is normally measured in degrees Celsius (°C). On this scale, water freezes at 0 °C and boils at 100 °C
- When measuring a temperature the choice of device and how the temperature is taken are both important
- Latent heat is the additional heat energy involved in changing the state of matter

- Sweating is important in controlling the body's core temperature
- Heat may be transmitted by conduction, convection and radiation
- Maintaining temperature homeostasis requires that heat losses from the body equal heat gains through metabolic processes
- Hypothermia and hyperthermia are extreme life-threatening conditions where the body's heat control mechanisms have ceased to be effective.

Review questions

12.1. Calculate the total heat loss from the body due to sweating $850\,cm^3$ water ($1\,cm^3$ water has a mass of $1\,g$, the latent heat of vaporisation of water is $2260\,kg^{-1}$).

12.2. Why is a clinical thermometer not suitable for measuring the ward temperature?

12.3. Look at the vacuum flask in Fig. 12.8. How does the design of this flask minimise the transmission of heat by:

   i) conduction
  ii) convection
 iii) radiation?

12.4. What precautions would you recommend to avoid the occurrence of hyperthermia in the aged?

Further reading

Marieb, E.N. (2000). *Human Anatomy and Physiology* 5th Edn. Benjamin Cummings, Redwood City, California.

Hickman, R. & Caon, M. (1995). *Nursing Science: Matter and Energy in the Human Body* 2nd Edn. Macmillan, Melbourne. Chapter 5.

Cree, L. & Rischmiller, S. (1995). *Science in Nursing* 3rd Edn. Baillière Tindall, London. Chapter 2.

Chapter Thirteen
FORCES AND MECHANICS

Learning objectives

By the end of this chapter the reader will be able to:
- Describe what is meant by forces
- State the laws that govern them
- Describe the significance of gravity as a force and the importance of the centre of gravity
- Explain how friction between surfaces is a resistance to movement
- Describe how the body (skeleton and limbs) acts as a system of levers that if used correctly can move objects safely and efficiently.

Introduction

Moving patients is one of the most important and potentially hazardous activities undertaken by nurses. This is borne out by the depressing statistics for back injuries in nurses, some of which lead to the termination of their careers. The Manual Handling Operations Regulations and the advent of more ergonomically sound approaches to moving and handling are important advances. To appreciate the principles behind these modern approaches we need to understand the ideas of force, centre of gravity, friction and levers.

Getting things moving – Newton's laws of motion

You will be familiar with the idea that to get an object moving you have to give it a push or a pull. In other words you will have to apply a force to the object.

Newton's first law of motion

This is the idea expressed in Newton's first law of motion 'that a body will continue at rest or in a state of uniform motion unless acted on by an unbalanced force'.

The direction in which the object moves will be the same as the direction of the applied force so the force is described as a vector as it has both magnitude and direction. We can represent the size and direction of the force by an arrow (Fig. 13.1). This idea may seem obvious but it is important when we look at the forces that resist the motion of objects.

An unfortunate consequence of Newton's first law is when you are thrown forward as a vehicle stops suddenly. The vehicle is stopped by application of its brakes or an impact but you continue moving in the same direction unless restrained or thrown against something immovable. Even if you are in a car seat and wearing a restraining seatbelt you are at risk of serious neck injury (whiplash) as your head is not restrained and is rapidly jerked forward and

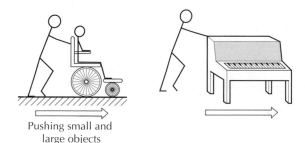

Pushing small and
large objects

Fig. 13.1 Pushing small and large objects.

then back with the likelihood of damage to the muscles and ligaments of the neck.

Car manufacturers have countered this problem with the introduction of airbags that will provide additional restraint in the event of impact. The inflated air bag cushions the head of the occupant and prevents the occupant hitting the dashboard, steering wheel or windscreen.

Newton's second law of motion

This tells us that the acceleration of an object (how quickly its speed increases) is proportional to the force applied to it.

This can be summarised by the equation:

force = mass × acceleration

The SI unit of force is the newton (named after Sir Isaac Newton of falling apple fame). A force of one newton applied to a mass of 1 kg will give it an acceleration of 1 metre per second (ms^{-1}).

This equation tells us that how quickly the object accelerates will depend on the mass of the object and the size of the force applied. The greater the mass of a body the greater the force required for the same amount of acceleration.

Think of the situation when you have to push a trolley or bed. When we start an object moving it will accelerate. We normally then allow it to move at a constant speed so it is no longer accelerating and the force we require for this is now less. In getting the object moving we have to overcome the inertia of the object.

Once that is overcome, the force required to keep it moving is reduced.

Work and energy

Remember that the work we do uses up the energy that we have available to get us through the day – we can make an estimate of this since:

$$\text{Work done} = \text{force applied} \times \text{distance moved by the object}$$

We measure work (and the energy required to achieve it) in joules (J) or kilojoules (kJ). It requires 1 joule of work to move an object 1 metre where the force needed is 1 newton.

In order to be efficient we need to consider both how far we have to move objects and also is the force we are applying fully effective in doing the work we require?

If we apply the force at an angle, as in the example of pushing the wheelchair (Fig. 13.2) the direction of the force we are applying is not totally in the direction that the wheelchair is able to travel. We can see that our applied force has a horizontal component (effective) and a vertical component (useless). The lesson to be learned is that the direction of the force should be as close to the direction of movement as possible. This may be achieved by changing our posture or adjusting the equipment.

You will know from pushing a bed or trolley that it will continue to move forward in a straight line and that turning corners will require an additional force in the new direction to change its course. This also illustrates the directional nature of a force.

Sometimes we push an object and it doesn't move! If that is the case then we have not overcome the inertia of the object (there is an opposite force that cancels out the one we are applying to the object).

This demonstrates another important principle – that of balanced forces. If an object is not moving we can deduce that the forces acting on it are all cancelling each other out. As we shall see below, the most significant forces that resist motion are those of gravity and friction.

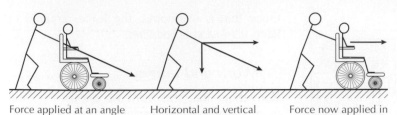

| Force applied at an angle | Horizontal and vertical components of a force | Force now applied in the direction of travel |

Fig. 13.2 Directional components of a force.

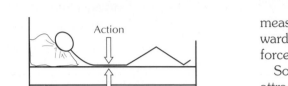

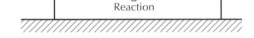

Fig. 13.3 'Action and reaction' – patient supported on a bed.

Newton's third law of motion

The third law of motion states that 'for every action there is an equal and opposite reaction' and helps to explain the idea of balanced forces mentioned above.

Think of a patient lying on a bed. We all recognise that the bed supports the patient, without the bed the patient would fall to the floor. The patient would fall because of the downward force of gravity. That the patient does not fall depends upon the bed pushing up with an equal and opposite force. The forces cancel each other out, the patient does not move up or down (Fig. 13.3).

The force of gravity

Before we go further we need to be clear about the difference between 'mass' and 'weight'. Mass is a measure of the amount of material in an object, nowadays usually measured in the SI units: grams (g) or kilograms (kg).

If we want to measure the mass of an object we use weighing scales. What we are actually measuring is the weight of the object – the downward force on the scales is due to the downward force of gravity on the object in question.

So, what is gravity? The force of gravity attracts any two bodies together. How large the force is depends on the size of the two bodies and how close they are to each other. The force of gravity between the earth and our body is sufficiently large to keep us from drifting away from the earth in weightlessness! The earth is massive so it attracts all objects towards its centre very strongly. In fact we experience an acceleration towards the centre of the earth of $9.81\,\mathrm{ms^{-2}}$ (metres per second squared). This is, of course, why Newton observed the apple falling downwards from the tree!

Compare this with the moon (about one sixth of the size of the earth) where the force of gravity is one sixth of that experienced on earth. This leads to the partial weightlessness experienced by astronauts who have tried walking on the moon. If you could distance yourself even further from the earth in a spaceship, you would experience virtually true weightlessness!

Back on earth, a body with a mass of 1 kg subjected to gravity's accelerating effects exerts a downward force of 9.81 newtons (refer to Table 13.1). (We use the approximation that 1 kg is approximately equivalent to 10 newtons.)

Centre of gravity

The centre of gravity of an object (or body) is a useful way of representing the effect of gravity. We can consider that the entire weight of the body can be seen to be acting through this point. The idea of the centre of gravity is impor-

Table 13.1 The effects of gravity

Nursing application	Explanation
IV drip bags suspended above patient	The force of gravity provides sufficient force to enable the introduction of solutions into veins (saline drips, blood transfusions)
Fluid drainage	When draining fluids from a patient you must ensure that there is downward drainage (so the bag is below the point of drainage from the patient's body) e.g. urine bags during catheterisation
Reduction of venous bleeding by raising limb	The heart has to pump blood 'uphill' against the force of gravity and the supply of blood is reduced
Procedure for improving blood circulation with a fainting patient	Laying a person flat and raising the legs will encourage the flow of blood to the brain which may have been partially starved of oxygen prior to the faint

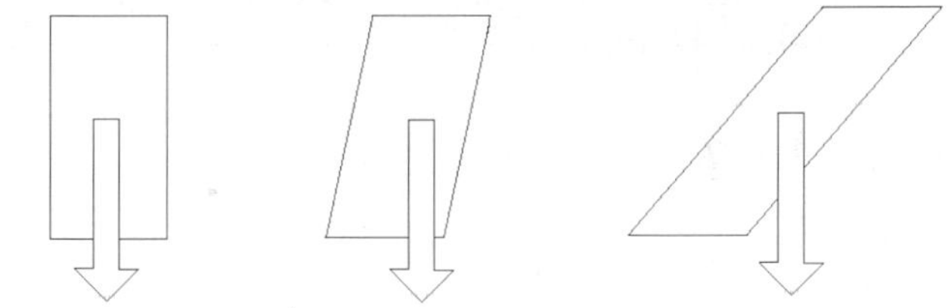

Stable body, centre of gravity falls in middle of base

Centre of gravity near edge of base; a small force will make object topple

Centre of gravity outside base; object falls immediately

Fig. 13.4 Centre of gravity.

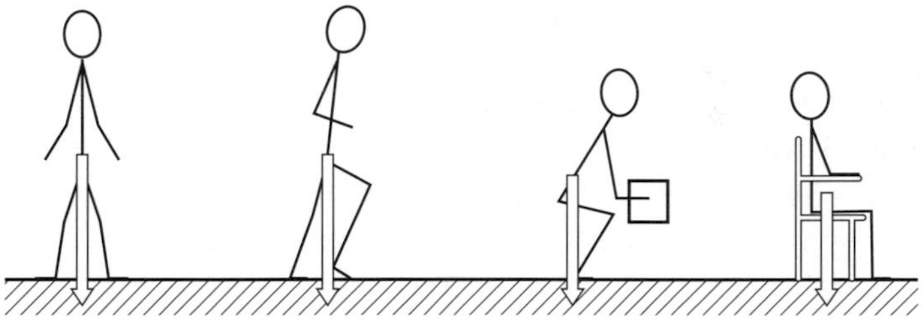

Fig. 13.5 Centre of gravity in various activities.

Centre of gravity of an erect adult (good posture)

Centre of gravity of a walker

Centre of gravity while lifting

Centre of gravity of a seated person

tant in understanding the stability of an object. If a vertical line drawn from the centre of gravity of the object lies within the base of the body, the object will be stable, if not it will have a tendency to topple over (Figs 13.4 and 13.5).

There are a number of situations in nursing where understanding the significance of the position of the centre of gravity is important.

These include:

- good posture in lifting situations
- ensuring stability for unstable patients.

In both cases the principle of providing a substantial base to support the body applies. Placing your feet apart during the lifting process ensures that the centre of gravity remains within the base you have created, removing the possibility of falling over. In addition, the nearer the centre of gravity remains to the centre of the 'base', the less is the strain on the spine and limbs of the body.

For stability when walking, the pelvis must shift to allow the centre of gravity to be above the grounded leg to allow the non weight-bearing leg to swing forward. Lack of pelvic control makes this a difficult operation!

The stability of aged or infirm patients can therefore be improved by the use of a walking frame, crutches or walking stick. In each case the walking aid widens the base of support and increases the safety of the patient whilst in motion (Fig. 13.6).

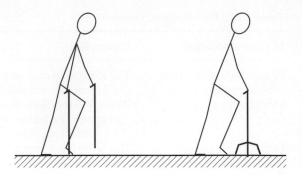

Fig. 13.6 Walking aids.

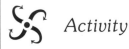 *Activity*

Some things you can do to illustrate the importance of the correct positioning of the centre of gravity, and the strain on your muscles if you do not:

- Stand upright with correct posture. Now lean forward. What do you feel?
- Stand balanced on one leg. Again what do you feel?
- Sit upright on a chair with your back against the rest. Try to get up from the chair without changing your body shape! Why is it difficult? (Referring to the position of the centre of gravity when seated will help!)
- Now try to get up in the normal way. How do you move your centre of gravity to enable you to rise from the chair?

Friction

Friction is the force that opposes the sliding of two surfaces, one over the other. The forces of friction are at times essential, in other situations they are a hindrance that we strive to overcome. In any situation where one surface moves over another, friction will play a part.

Friction between surfaces arises because no two surfaces in contact are completely smooth (even when polished) and the rough nature of the surfaces causes them to interlock to a greater or lesser extent (Fig. 13.7).

Without the effects of friction we would not be able to walk as the grip between footwear and the floor is essential – hence the importance of avoiding slippery floors in hospitals! Friction between surfaces is reduced by the lubricating effects of liquid (remember that the molecules of a liquid slide over each other easily) so spillages of liquids increase the likelihood of harmful slips.

Friction also produces wear as the interlocking surfaces interact with each other and are damaged, rough surfaces tend to become smoother with time.

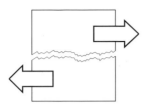

Fig. 13.7 Friction between objects caused by interlocking surfaces.

Reducing the effects of friction

Where we want surfaces to slide over each other easily, friction is a negative factor. Unwanted resistance to motion and wear can result from this effect.

The use of wheels is the most common way of reducing the effects of friction. Compare sliding an object along the floor and using a trolley with wheels to move the same object. The 'drag' due to friction is massively reduced (Fig. 13.8).

Lubrication is another way of overcoming unwanted friction, examples of this include:

* Inside the body, mucus (lungs, heart and intestines) and saliva (digesting food) are essential body lubricants
* Synovial fluid reduces friction and wear between cartilage in synovial joints
* Use of lubricants (e.g. K–Y jelly®) during the insertion of instruments and catheters into the body
* If the downward force on an object sliding over another is increased, the frictional force is also increased – hence the use of skin lotions and oils during massage.

With the increase in the use of horizontal transfers rather than the lifting of patients in nursing, equipment such as sliding sheets, banana boards and transfer boards have become commonplace as ward equipment (Fig. 13.9). These 'sliding' techniques rely on the use of low friction surfaces to enable the patient to be transferred relatively effortlessly (only a small force is required to induce the sliding) by the carer(s) or themselves.

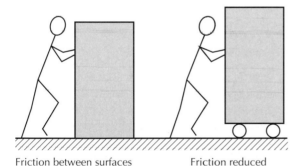

Friction between surfaces   Friction reduced

Fig. 13.8 Reducing friction.

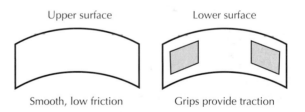

Upper surface   Lower surface

Smooth, low friction   Grips provide traction

Fig. 13.9 The banana board.

✺ Activity

Investigate the design and the materials used in the manufacture of sliding sheets.

The avoidance of pressure sores

An important aspect of caring for bedridden patients is to take steps to ensure that pressure sores do not develop. These sores can develop by a combination of the localisation of the forces of action and reaction, which have been described above, and the effects of friction.

Remember that pressure at a particular point is dependent on both the force and the area over which that force is applied. If we increase the area then for a given force the pressure is reduced as the force is spread over a wider area. This is expressed by the equation:

$$\text{Pressure} = \frac{\text{Force}}{\text{Area}}$$

A favourite illustration of this is to compare the not dissimilar pressure exerted by a standing elephant (with four broad feet to

---

Exercise 13.1

Which exerts the greater downward pressure?
   A weight of 70 kg supported on a base of 0.01 m² (square metres) or 700 kg spread over 0.1 m²? (Assume a weight of 1 kg exerts a downward force of 10 newtons).

---

spread the load) with a woman wearing stiletto heels!

Pressure sores are believed to result from the sustained effect of pressure on the skin which restricts the capillary blood flow beneath the skin. This causes cell death and subsequent ulceration. The friction between patient and bedding then further exacerbates this situation. When the patient is lying down it is easy to see that the forces acting on the skin are localised at the points of contact between the patient and the bed (Fig. 13.10), in particular the bony areas.

Consequently, the first principle of avoiding pressure sores is keeping the patient mobile to vary the points of contact between patient and bed. If patient mobility is restricted then pressure relieving cushions, mattresses or beds may have to be employed. Whatever method is employed the principle must be to reduce the prolonged pressure at particular points on the skin by either varying the points of contact or reducing pressure by spreading the overall load of the body.

Levers

A lever is a simple mechanical device (machine) that enables us to apply a force at one point and see its effect at another. Our limbs are used as levers when we move and when we carry objects. The simplest illustration of a lever is a seesaw (Fig. 13.11). Looking at how this works will enable us to understand the terms involved and how more complex levers work.

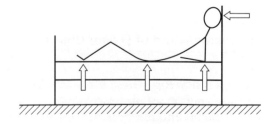

Fig. 13.10 Localisation of pressure sores.

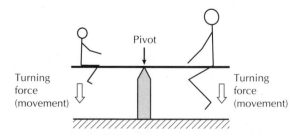

Fig. 13.11 Turning forces on a see-saw.

When a force rotates an object about a pivot (as in the see-saw) the magnitude of the turning force (or moment) increases with the size of the force and the distance from the turning point (or pivot). The turning force is calculated by multiplying the force by the distance from the pivot:

$$\text{Turning force (moment)} = \text{applied force} \times \text{distance from pivot}$$

A force of one newton placed 1 m from the pivot gives a turning force of 1 newton metre (Nm).

As the equation indicates the greater the distance between the point where the force is applied and the pivot, the greater is the applied moment. So, by increasing the distance we can produce a greater turning force with the same applied force – we have a useful machine!

Load and effort

For two people to balance on the see-saw it is necessary for the turning force produced by each person (one considered to be the load, the other the effort) to be equal and opposite so they cancel out:

$$\text{Load} \times \text{distance of load from pivot} = \text{effort} \times \text{distance of effort from pivot}$$

If the two people occupying the see-saw are of differing weights the lighter one will need to sit at a point further from the pivot for the balance to occur. You will no doubt be familiar with this from your playground experiences but you can check it out by balancing a ruler at its mid-point and loading it with different weights at either end, moving them until they come to balance each other.

 ## Exercise 13.2

A father and his child are trying to balance a see-saw. The father (60 kg) sits close to the pivot (1 m away). The child (30 kg) sits at the opposite end, making her 2 m away from the pivot. Calculate the turning forces to see whether they will achieve their objective!

Mechanical advantage

The see-saw example shows that moving the position where the effort is applied further away from the pivot offers the opportunity of lifting a larger load than the effort being put in. We say that the machine has a mechanical advantage.

Remember that on a balanced see-saw the product of the load and its distance from the pivot is equal to the product of the effort and its distance from the pivot:

$$\text{Load} \times \text{distance of load from pivot} = \text{effort} \times \text{distance of effort from pivot}$$

If we rearrange that equation we come up with the expression:

$$\frac{\text{Load}}{\text{Effort}} = \frac{\text{distance of effort from pivot}}{\text{distance of load from pivot}}$$

This ratio of load over effort is called the mechanical advantage. If the load is greater than the effort that is provided then the mechanical advantage is more than one; if the effort is greater than the load, the mechanical advantage is less than one.

The see-saw is an example of a 1st order lever. Examples of 1st, 2nd and 3rd order levers in the human body are given in Table 13.2.

Table 13.2 Types of lever

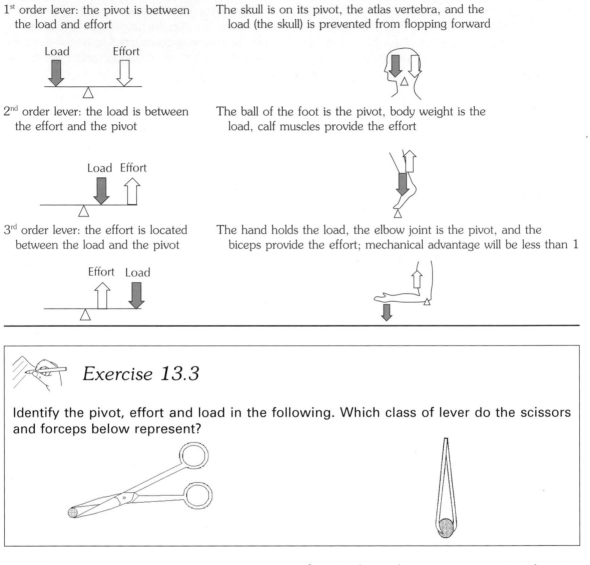

1st order lever: the pivot is between the load and effort	The skull is on its pivot, the atlas vertebra, and the load (the skull) is prevented from flopping forward
2nd order lever: the load is between the effort and the pivot	The ball of the foot is the pivot, body weight is the load, calf muscles provide the effort
3rd order lever: the effort is located between the load and the pivot	The hand holds the load, the elbow joint is the pivot, and the biceps provide the effort; mechanical advantage will be less than 1

Exercise 13.3

Identify the pivot, effort and load in the following. Which class of lever do the scissors and forceps below represent?

Pulleys

Pulleys are also simple machines. They may be fixed or moveable pulleys as illustrated in Fig. 13.12. A fixed pulley simply allows you to change the direction of a force that is applied. A moveable pulley also offers some mechanical advantage as the effort moves further than the load.

Pulleys find applications in traction and hoists. In both cases the direction of the applied force is changed to a more convenient direction (Fig. 13.13).

Forces, levers and moving and handling issues

To complete the chapter, let us look at how we can apply the principles of levers to explain some aspects of moving and handling.

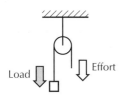
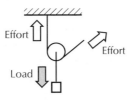

Fixed pulley   Moveable pulley

Fig. 13.12 Pulleys.

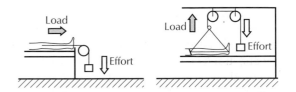

Fig. 13.13 Traction and hoist.

Holding the load close to the body

One of the first things you are taught in relation to moving and handling is that you must keep the load as close to the body as possible whilst lifting (Fig. 13.14). Applying the principles of levers we can now see why the further a load is held from the body the heavier it appears to be.

With a load held at arm's length the distance between the load and the pivot (shoulder) is substantial and the turning forces produced are significant. By holding the load close to the body the distance is reduced significantly, consequently so are the turning forces.

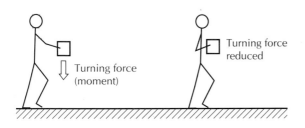

Fig. 13.14 Holding the load close to the body.

Adopting the correct posture

When lifting you are instructed to keep your spine straight and rigid and that the effort for lifting should come from your thigh muscles. If this advice is followed, in lever terms the hip joint becomes the pivot and we have an example of a third class lever (Fig. 13.15).

If however you allow the spine to become the pivot (Fig. 13.16), substantial turning forces are exerted on the spine's vertebrae and discs, pos-

sibly leading to herniation – a 'slipped disc'. The effort to support and raise the load is provided by the muscle groups at the base of the spine that may also be injured as a result.

Horizontal transfers

Current moving and handling practice is based on the principle of horizontal rather than vertical transfer of patients. Vertical transfers of patients (where the patient must be lifted)

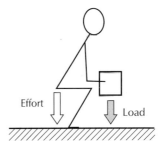

Fig. 13.15 Lifting from the hip.

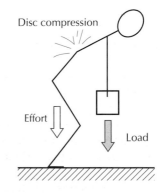
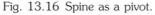

Fig. 13.16 Spine as a pivot.

should employ the use of mechanised pulleys (hoists) since the loads to be lifted are considered too large to be lifted safely by staff. Sliding sheets, transfer boards and similar equipment are used to carry out horizontal transfers wherever possible. In doing so the forces that the nurse is required to apply are reduced by:

- avoiding working against the effect of gravity which has to be overcome when lifting objects
- minimising the frictional forces which oppose horizontal motion.

Not only does this reduce risk of injury but also it reduces the overall physical workload of the carer throughout the working day. Remember this when some staff criticise the introduction of these modern working practices!

Summary

- Forces are required to get objects moving. They are vector quantities and have both magnitude and direction
- Newton's three laws of motion describe how objects behave under the influence of a force:
  - Force is required to get bodies moving
  - The rate of acceleration will be dependent on the size of the force and mass of the object
  - Every force induces an equal and opposite reaction
- The force of gravity causes all bodies to be attracted (accelerated) towards the centre of the earth; this means there is a downward force on our bodies
- For an object to be stable, the centre of gravity should lie within the base of the object
- Friction is a resistance to motion when two surfaces are in contact; lubrication or low friction materials will reduce this effect

- Levers are simple machines that allow the effect of a force to be felt at a point other than its application
- The turning force about a pivot increases with the distance between the load or force and the pivot
- A mechanical advantage can be achieved by the appropriate design of lever or pulley systems.

Review questions

13.1.   You are wheeling a trolley along a corridor. Only a small force is needed to keep the trolley moving. You come to a corner and you find that more force is needed to get it round the corner. Explain these two observations.

13.2.   Explain why we are told that our feet should provide a wide base whilst lifting.

13.3.   Two solids objects sliding over each other will be subject to significant frictional forces. The introduction of a liquid between the surfaces will reduce the friction. Use what you know about the properties of liquids to explain this observation.

13.4   Holding a box at arm's length is more tiring than holding it close to your body. Explain!

Rurther reading

Mariab, E.N. (2000). *Human Anatomy and Physiology* (5th edn). Benjamin Cummings, Redwood City, California.

Hickman, R. & Caon, M. (1995). *Nursing Science: Matter and Energy in the Human Body* (2nd edn). Macmillan, Melbourne.

Manual Handling: Guidance on Regulations (L23) 1998. HSE Books, Sudbury.

Cree, L. & Rischmiller, S. (1995). *Science in Nursing* (3rd edn). Baillière Tindall, London.

The Guide to the Handling of Patients (4th edn). 1998. NBPA, Teddington.

Chapter Fourteen
ELECTRICITY

Learning objectives

By the end of this chapter the reader will be able to:
- Distinguish between static and dynamic (current) electricity
- Define the terms potential difference, current, resistance and power and be able to give units for each
- Discuss the effects of electrocution and differentiate between macroshock and microshock
- Know how to use electricity safely
- Describe how nerve impulses are transmitted and how the conduction system of the heart works
- Briefly describe medical applications of electricity.

Introduction

Electricity is an essential part of our modern society. At home we use electricity to watch television or listen to music on our stereos, in hospitals medical equipment and machinery are powered by electricity. Our bodies use electricity to transmit nerve impulses and make muscles contract – life could not exist without electricity.

However, electricity can kill and from an early age we are taught the dangers of electricity and how to use it safely. In this chapter we will look at the medical applications of electricity and how to minimise the risks involved in its use.

Electricity

Electricity is the flow or movement of electrons – electrons are negatively charged particles found in all atoms. Substances that allow the flow of electrons are called conductors. All metals are good conductors of electricity, e.g. copper and aluminium. Insulators do not allow

the flow of electrons. Examples of insulators are rubber, plastics, ceramics, wood and glass. The myelin sheath of the neurones (nerve cells) is a good insulator and prevents electrical conduction between neurones and their surroundings (see Fig. 14.6 later). If the myelin sheath becomes damaged or destroyed problems occur with the conduction of nerve impulses, multiple sclerosis is an example of one such disease. There are two forms of electricity – static and dynamic (current) electricity.

Static electricity

As the name suggests in static electricity there is a build-up of electrons in one place. Static electricity is caused by friction or the rubbing together of two insulators. As the materials are rubbed together, electrons are 'pulled off' one substance and 'dumped' on the other. This causes a build-up of electrons resulting in a negative charge on one material and a loss of electrons in the other material, giving a positive charge. The direction of transfer of electrons depends on the materials being used (Fig. 14.1).

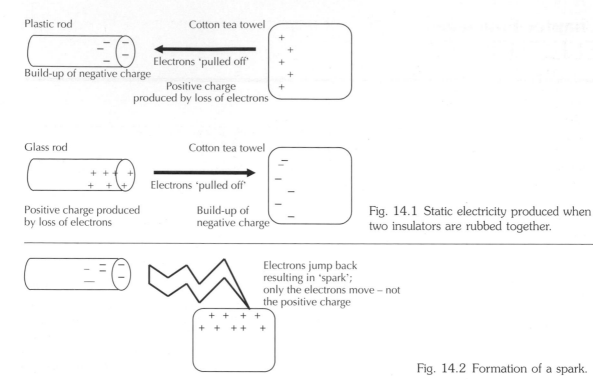

Fig. 14.1 Static electricity produced when two insulators are rubbed together.

Fig. 14.2 Formation of a spark.

As the number of electrons build up so does the charge. The charge is eventually removed when the electrons 'jump' back to a region with an opposite charge causing a spark, or shock (Fig. 14.2). This shows that there are two types of charge, positive (+) and negative (−) and that like charges repel but unlike charges attract. Lightning is an example of the movement of electrons, from the clouds to earth.

A nurse may encounter static electricity when making a bed. The bed is insulated by rubber tyres and a build-up of charge occurs. When the nurse touches the bed the electrons are transferred to the nurse and earthed giving the nurse a shock. For this reason, cotton blankets are preferred to woollen or polyester, since both the latter build up more static electricity. In operating theatres static electricity can be a source of ignition in anaesthetic explosions, thus loose fitting cotton clothing is preferred and special antistatic footwear is worn. Also, modern operating theatres are designed to prevent the build-

---

✣ Activity

Try the following activities to demonstrate static electricity:
a)   Blow up a balloon. Rub the balloon against your jumper. TAKE CARE! The balloon should now stick to your jumper or to the wall thanks to static electricity.
b)   Comb your hair with a plastic comb then pick up small pieces of paper with the comb.
c)   Buy some really cheap and nasty nylon underwear, petticoat or vest. Wear a woolly jumper. When undressing turn out the light and watch the sparks fly.
Will these activities work better in humid or dry conditions?

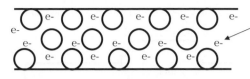

Fig. 14.3 Conduction in metals.

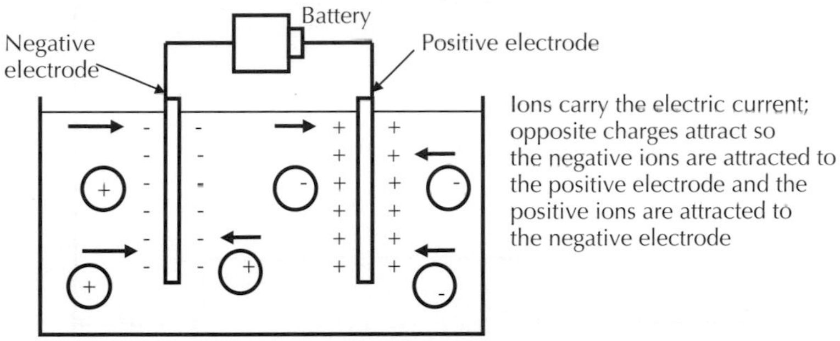

Sea of electrons (e-)
carry current.

Negative
electrode

Battery

Positive electrode

Ions carry the electric current;
opposite charges attract so
the negative ions are attracted to
the positive electrode and the
positive ions are attracted to
the negative electrode

Fig. 14.4 Conduction in
electrolytes.

up of static electricity with special floors and equipment.

Dynamic (current) electricity

Dynamic electricity involves the flow of either electrons or ions. The flow of these electrons and ions results in an electrical current. In metals the current is carried only by electrons. Metals contain a 'sea of electrons' which are free to carry the electrical current (Fig. 14.3). This is why metals are such good conductors. Electrolytes such as sodium chloride are substances that produce negative and positive ions in solution and both these ions carry the current (Fig. 14.4). Electrical currents in the body are carried by ions.

Pure water is a poor conductor under normal conditions. However, the addition of electrolytes to water makes it a good conductor. For this reason saline (sodium chloride in water) or tap water which contains various electrolytes are good conductors.

Potential difference and current

The potential difference is the difference in charge between two points. Electrons will only flow from an area where they are in high con-

centration to an area where they are in low concentration. The greater the difference in electron concentration (charge) between two points, the greater the potential difference. The flow of electrons from one point to another generates an electrical current (I). The greater the size of the potential difference the greater the current. The unit of current is the ampere or amp (A). The potential difference is therefore the driving force that pushes the current around, it is a kind of electrical pressure. The unit of measure for potential difference is the volt (V). The potential difference or voltage of the domestic mains supply is 240 V and a car battery is 12 V. In the body potential differences occur across all cell membranes. Since the potential differences in the body are usually very small the millivolt (mV) is used, e.g. depending on the cell and organism the resting cell potential is between −20 to −200 mV. For a current to flow there must be a complete path or circuit for it to flow around (Fig. 14.5).

Resistance

Resistance is the opposition to the flow of electrons and its unit is the ohm (Ω). (Fig. 14.5). Metals, such as copper, silver and aluminium are all good conductors, since they offer less

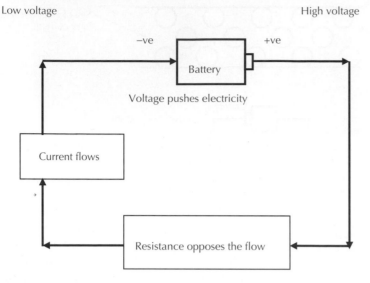

Fig. 14.5 Circuit diagram.

resistance to electron flow than other substances. Solids are normally better conductors than liquids and liquids better conductors than gases. Gases tend to be insulators due to their lack of charge.

Resistance of a material depends on:

- Temperature – high temperatures increase resistance, since electrons undergo a larger number of collisions
- Length of conductor – the longer the conductor, the greater the resistance
- Purity of conductor – the purer the conductor, the less the resistance
- Thickness of conductor – the thicker the wire, the less the resistance.

In the body the skin, bones and oil secreted by the sebaceous glands all provide resistance to the flow of electricity. For this reason special gels are used to lower skin resistance when electricity is being used diagnostically, e.g. electrocardiogram (ECG). Cleaning the skin (e.g. with alcohol wipes) also helps to lower skin resistance.

Fuses are pieces of resistance wire that are added to circuits to act as 'safety valves'. If a large current is sent through the circuit the fuse melts and blows and so breaks the circuit, preventing the flow of electricity. However, the current needed to blow a fuse is still large enough to kill a person.

The relationship between current, voltage and resistance is given by Ohm's law.

$$\text{Current (A)} = \frac{\text{Voltage (V)}}{\text{Resistance (Ohm)}} \text{ or } I = \frac{V}{R}$$

As can be seen from the above equation, the greater the potential difference (voltage) the greater the current, and the greater the resistance the smaller the current.

Power

Power is the rate at which energy is changed into work, i.e. the rate at which electricity is consumed in a given time. The unit of power is the watt (W) and it can be calculated as follows:

power = voltage × current
(watts)　(volts)　(amps)

The watt is a small unit so the kilowatt (kW) is used (1000 watt = 1 kilowatt).

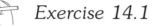

Exercise 14.1

How much current does a 60 watt electric light bulb use on a 240 V mains supply?

Direct and alternating current

Direct current (dc) is current that travels in one direction only. Direct current is needed for most electronic appliances (e.g. TVs, computers and monitors). Alternating current (ac) is current that changes its direction back and forth. Mains electricity is ac with a frequency of 50 Hz (Hz = cycle per second), which means it reverses direction 50 times every second. Dynamos and power stations produce alternating current. Only alternating current can be used in transformers. Transformers are able to change the voltage to suit various electrical appliances, e.g. electric blankets, shavers.

Electricity and the body

Mechanism of nerve impulses

The nervous system is made up of specialised cells called neurones (can also be spelt as neurons) or nerve cells (Fig. 14.6). Neurones transmit messages very rapidly in a series of electrical changes known as a nerve impulse or action potential. Neurones conduct nerve impulses due to the changes in the potential difference across the cell membrane.

Resting membrane potential

A 'resting' neurone is one that is not conducting a nerve impulse. However, a potential difference still exists across the cell membrane. Extracellular fluid normally contains about 10 sodium ions for every potassium ion. Inside the cell this position is reversed. The cell membrane of a neurone is relatively impermeable to

sodium but permeable to potassium. Thus, there is a slow inflow of sodium and an outflow of potassium by diffusion. The sodium/potassium pump also transports three sodium ions out of the cell for every two potassium ions it brings into the cell. This requires energy in the form of ATP. However the potassium ions that are pumped in diffuse back out. The net effect of these two processes is to make the outer surface of the axon membrane positive and the inner surface of the axon membrane negative. In these conditions there is a potential difference across the membrane of around −70 mV (the negative sign indicates that the inside is negative relative to the outside). The potential difference across the membrane at rest is the

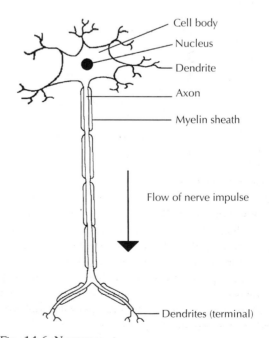

Fig. 14.6 Neurone.

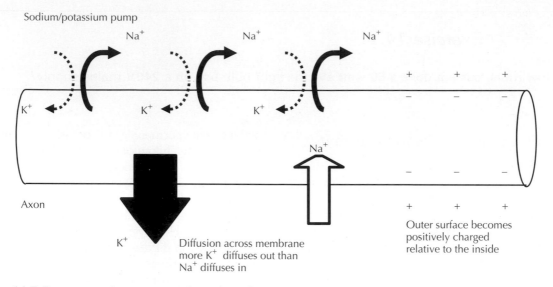

Fig. 14.7 Resting membrane potential – polarised.

resting membrane potential and the membrane is said to be polarised (Fig. 14.7).

The sodium/potassium pump stabilises the resting membrane potential by providing a diffusion gradient for the sodium and potassium ions.

The action potential

The stimulation of a neurone results in a change in the potential difference across the axon membrane. The negative value of −70 mV inside the cell becomes briefly positive at +40 mV. This reversal of membrane potential is called an action potential and it results in the transmission of an impulse. The key to the change in polarity is that on stimulation the permeability of the membrane alters. The action potential is generated by the brief opening of the ion channels in the membrane called sodium gates. Sodium rushes into the cell making the inside of the membrane positive rather than negative. The neurone is now said to be depolarised (Fig. 14.8).

Return to resting potential

Shortly after depolarisation the sodium gates close and the potassium gates open. Potassium diffuses out of the neurone and at the same time, the sodium/potassium pump also moves sodium ions out of the neurone and potassium ions in. This makes the inside of the cell relatively less positive or more negative – the start of repolarisation and the return to the original resting potential (Fig. 14.9). Therefore, the resting potential is determined largely by potassium ions, but the action potential is determined largely by sodium ions.

There is in fact a slight 'overshoot' into a more negative potential than the original resting membrane potential value – this is called hyperpolarisation and is due to the slight delay in closing all the potassium gates compared to the sodium gates. The overshoot is corrected by the sodium/potassium pump (Fig. 14.10).

There is a very short time interval, less than a millisecond, when another action potential cannot be generated. This is the refractory period and it ensures that the impulse moves in

Sodium gates open and sodium moves into cell

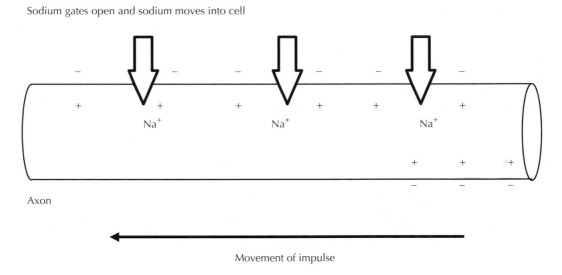

Axon

Movement of impulse

Fig. 14.8 Action potential – depolarisation.

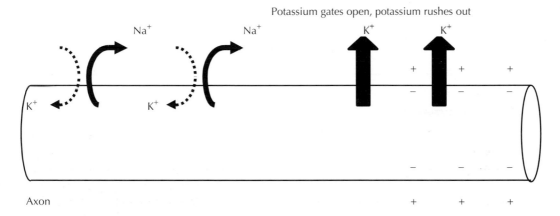

Potassium gates open, potassium rushes out

Axon

Fig. 14.9 Return to resting membrane potential – repolarisation.

a forward direction only. However neurones are still able to transmit about 500 impulses a second.

Propagation

Once generated the action potential needs to move along the length of the axon as a nerve impulse. In order to do this the action potential must be propagated (sent or transmitted). Propagation occurs due to the effect of sodium ions entering the axon. The sodium ions generate an area of positive charge and current can flow in a local circuit set up between this active positive area and the negatively charged resting area of the axon immediately ahead. The local current flow depolarises the adjacent membrane and this results in the sodium gates opening and the generation of a new action potential. Repeated depolarisation results in the action potential being moved or propagated along the axon (Fig. 14.11).

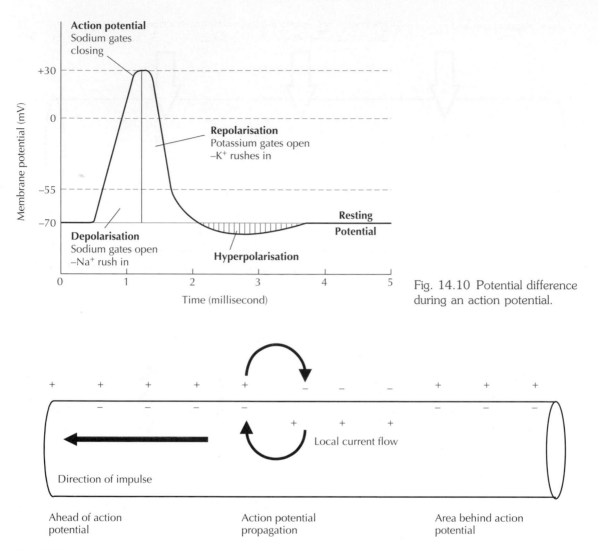

Fig. 14.10 Potential difference during an action potential.

Fig. 14.11 Propagation.

The conduction system of the heart

The heart beats 70 beats per minute at rest, 100 000 beats a day or 1.825×10^9 beats during a 50-year life span. The heart beats continuously due to its electrical properties. The cardiac muscle action potential is similar to that of a neurone but lasts much longer. The contraction of the heart is initiated within the heart at the sinoatrial node (SA node). The SA node sets the heart rate and so is known as the pacemaker. Unlike skeletal muscle the heart does not require any stimulation from the nervous system to contract. The stimulation for each heart beat comes from the heart itself and is intrinsic and its characteristic rhythm is called the sinus rhythm. Due to this a heart will beat happily outside the body for an hour or more without any outside stimulus.

Shortly after leaving the SA node the electrical impulse reaches the atrioventricular node

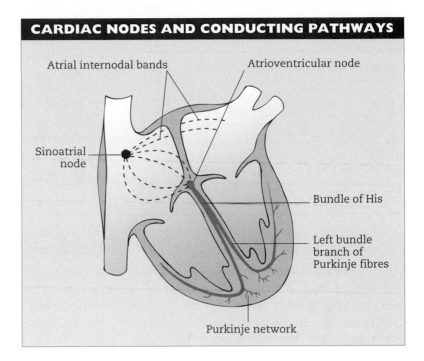

Fig. 14.12 The intrinsic conduction system of the heart.

(AV node). The AV node slows the conduction of the impulse allowing the atria to finish contracting before the ventricles contract. From the AV node the impulse passes more rapidly through the bundle of His which divides into a branch for each ventricle. On reaching the apex of each ventricle the conducting system divides into tiny specialised cardiac muscle fibres called the Purkinje fibres. This arrangement allows the impulse to pass down a definite pathway and to all areas of the heart (Fig. 14.12).

Artificial pacemakers

Defects in the conducting system of the heart can result in arrhythmias (irregular heart beat), fibrillation (unco-ordinated, chaotic beating or quivering of heart muscle) and heart block. A defect in the pacemaking SA node results in a slower than normal heart beat (bradycardia), e.g. sick sinus syndrome, however the impulses will still travel through the heart. When there is damage to the AV node, few or no impulses can pass from the atria to the ventricles and heart block occurs. In this case artificial pacemakers are used. In artificial pacemakers a battery powered pulse generator is implanted subcutaneously. The pulse reaches the heart through a wire passed into the right ventricle of the heart. There are two types of pacemaker:

- Fixed rate – the pacemaker delivers an impulse at constant rate to the heart
- Demand mode – the most common pacemaker today, which only works when the heart is not transmitting its own impulses. Patients with demand mode pacemakers may experience interference from external sources of electromagnetic radiation, e.g. security devices in airports.

Electrocution

When a body becomes part of an electrical circuit, the passage of current through the body can lead to death by electrocution. How electricity kills is still not exactly known but it is thought that it produces muscle contraction. The contraction of muscles leads to a 'can't let

Table 14.1 Effect of domestic electricity (50 Hz) on the body

Current mA (milliamps)	Effect on body
0.1	microshock fibrillation
0.5	threshold of sensation through skin
1.0	painful sensation
10–20	muscle spasm
greater than 100	ventricular fibrillation leading to cardiac arrest
greater than 1000	muscle burns

go' effect where the person being electrocuted is unable to break the circuit. The respiratory muscles also contract, preventing the person from breathing and the heart muscle contracts preventing blood flow to the body. Electrocution causes cardiac arrest, generally from ventricular fibrillation. Burns are also produced at the site of entry and exit of the body, the degree of burns will vary depending on the current.

The amount of damage done to the body depends on many factors:

- Amount of current – the major factor. Small currents of 1–5 mA will give shocks, sustained currents of 30–200 mA will lead to death (Table 14.1).
- Potential difference or voltage – the voltage is only important in the fact that it is sufficient to drive the current through the body.
- Path of current – small currents over large areas are not felt as much as the same current over smaller areas, e.g. a current passing through the body may result in ventricular fibrillation, however the same current passing through just a finger would cause burns. The current per unit area is known as current density, and the greater the current density the greater the heating effect.
- Frequency – the domestic mains supply has a frequency of 50 Hz. The heart is particularly sensitive to this frequency. Higher frequencies, as used in diathermy, are more

likely to burn the patient than cause muscle contraction.
- Resistance – the electrical resistance of the body can vary considerably. Dry skin is roughly 1000 times more resistant to a current than wet skin. So remember to dry your hands before turning on electrical equipment since with the same potential difference a greater current will be experienced by a person with wet skin.
- Duration of current – the longer the current flows the greater is the effect on the body.

Electric shock

In a hospital situation two types of shock are seen – macroschock and microshock. Macroshocks occur via electrical contact with the skin surface. The current passes through the entire body and there is no direct contact between the source of the current and the heart. Macroshock is the type of shock experienced by people in the home or at work and is the most common type of shock. In microshock, current flows directly to the heart without passing through the rest of the body.

One example where microshock can occur is when a transvenous pacing wire is in place as a temporary pacemaker. Here a pacemaker wire is passed through the vein directly into the right ventricle of the heart, the other end of the wire remains outside the body and is attached to a pacemaker box. In this situation very low currents, below the threshold of skin sensation, will cause ventricular fibrillation since any resistance provided by the body is bypassed (Table 14.1).

A nurse should attempt to avoid the generation of a circuit which includes the patient, e.g. do not touch the patient and another piece of electrical equipment through which a current could be conducted.

Electrical safety

Most electrocutions and electrical injuries are caused by a defective product, human error or

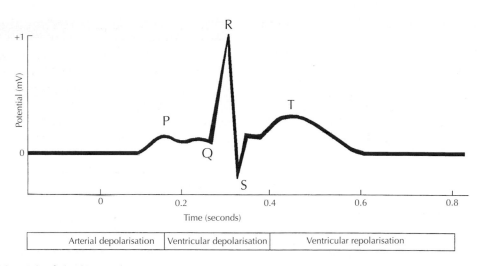

Fig. 14.13 ECG of the heart when at rest.

violation of local health and safety policies. All hospitals and other workplaces should have a health and safety policy which covers electrical safety, and you should familiarise yourself with these The following are some general guidelines:

- Water and electricity do not mix
- Plugs should be fitted with the correct fuse and wired correctly
- All electrical equipment should be tested periodically – different hospitals will have different policies
- Prevent microshock by wearing correct clothing, etc.
- Operate all equipment in accordance with manufacturer's instructions

- Check electrical appliances for wear and tear and report any defects to the appropriate staff
- All repairs must be carried out by a qualified electrician.

Medical applications of electricity

Electrocardiogram (ECG)

The electrical activity of the heart can be easily measured using an instrument called an electrocardiograph (the trace is called an electrocardiogram). A normal ECG consists of three waves called deflection waves (Fig. 14.13). Elec-

---

Exercise 14.2

Using Fig. 14.13 answer the following questions:
a)   How long is a single heart beat?
b)   How many heart beats are there in a minute?
c)   How much slower is conduction in the heart (Fig. 14.13) compared with conduction in a nerve impulse (Fig. 14.10)?

trocardiograms are used as diagnostic tools in hospitals since the size, frequency and duration of the waves seen are normally constant for a healthy person. Any change in the wave pattern can indicate underlying problems, e.g. heart block is seen as a P-wave which is not followed by a QRS complex; a lost P-wave indicates that the AV node has become the pacemaker and ventricular fibrillation would be seen as irregular chaotic waves.

Electroencephalogram (EEG)

An EEG is a way of measuring electrical patterns at the surface of the scalp by using electrodes. These patterns reflect the electrical activity of the brain – brainwaves. EEGs are frequently used to detect areas of brain damage by locating areas where wave patterns have changed. Its clinical use is mainly in the diagnosis of epilepsy, brain death, brain tumour and in sleep research.

Brainwaves occur at various frequencies – some are quick, some are slow. The four distinct wave patterns in the brain are:

- Alpha – (8–10 Hz) quick. Alpha waves occur with eyes closed and represent a relaxed or 'not doing much' state. Alpha disappears when person becomes mentally busy or on becoming drowsy
- Beta – (5–10 Hz) – small and quick, mentally alert and stimulated
- Delta – (1–2 Hz) – slow, deep sleep and in infants, brain damage
- Theta – (4–6 Hz) – slow, sleep.

Sleep

There are two types of sleep patterns, slow wave (SW) and rapid eye movement (REM) and we all spend our sleep cycling between these two states. EEG has detected at least four separate stages of sleep (Fig. 14.14).

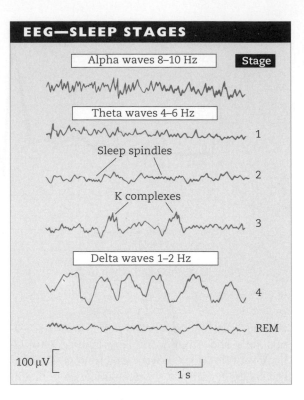

Fig. 14.14 EEG – sleep patterns.

Slow-wave sleep (SW)

During drowsiness, first alpha waves disappear and the size of theta waves increases. This is stage 1 of sleep. As sleep gets deeper (judged by how quickly a person wakes up) bursts of fast waves called 'sleep spindles' are seen – stage 2 of sleep. Stage 3 is characterised by high-amplitude delta waves and the presence of K complexes. Stage 4 consists of almost entirely large slow delta waves. During SW sleep there are reduced eye movement and muscle tone.

Rapid eye movement (REM)

During sleep the EEG shows desynchronised patterns resembling that recorded when the person is awake – eyes also move rapidly – this is REM sleep. It is more difficult to wake a person in REM sleep than SW sleep and REM sleep is accompanied by a number of signs of stress and excitement, e.g. irregularity in respiration, variation in blood pressure and pulse, penile erections and dreams. SW sleep appears to be necessary for body repair, whilst REM sleep is used to recover from mental fatigue.

Transcutaneous electrical nerve stimulation (TENS)

TENS can be used for the relief of pain in a large number of conditions. These include rheumatism, sciatica, back pain and whilst in labour. The TENS unit consists of a small battery, or electrical unit, and has electrode pads. These pads are placed around the pain site, and when in use the patient feels a tingling similar to 'pins and needles'. It is thought it works by 'closing the gate' for the transmission of pain from small nerve fibres by stimulating larger nerve fibres. This blocks the passage of pain messages to the brain and increases blood flow to the painful area. TENS also appears to stimulate the production of the body's own painkillers – endorphins. The effectiveness of TENS varies from patient to patient so the degree of pain relief wanted can be adjusted. TENS must never be used by anybody with a heart problem, pacemaker or in pregnancy (first trimester).

Defibrillator

The defibrillator is used for the treatment of ventricular fibrillation (uncoordinated, chaotic beating of the heart that may lead to a myocardial infarction – heart attack). Ventricular fibrillation is stopped by giving a large electrical shock via a defibrillator. The hope is that the shock will stop the heart twitching by depolarising the entire heart, allowing the SA node to start functioning properly again.

In a defibrillator electrical charge is stored and released in a controlled fashion. Many work-places, aeroplanes and all hospitals have defibrillators and trained operators should know where they are kept. The key component of a defibrillator is the capacitor – a device for storing charge. The capacitor can be charged from the mains or from an internal battery, and when not in use the defibrillator should be plugged into the mains. The capacitor should only be powered just before the unit is used.

To treat a patient the two electrodes or paddles are placed on the patient's chest at the base and over the apex of the heart. Both paddles have switches and both switches have to be pressed before a charge is delivered. If the patient is undergoing heart surgery sterile paddles can be used and a smaller charge delivered.

Diathermy

Diathermy involves passing a high frequency alternating current (typically 1 MHz or 1000 Hz) through the body (Fig. 14.15). The purpose of diathermy is to cut (electrosurgery) and seal blood vessels (electrocautery). Remember that nerves and the heart are most sensitive to low frequencies (50 Hz) so they are a not affected by the high frequency of diathermy.

In monopolar diathermy there are two electrodes, a large neutral patient plate or indifferent electrode and the smaller active electrode or diathermy probe used by the surgeon for cutting and sealing. The same current flows through both electrodes – however the narrow diathermy probe held by the surgeon results in heating and burning due to its large resistance. No burning should occur at the patient plate as the current flows through a very large area with little resistance. If the area of contact between patient and plate is reduced, burns may result to the patient.

Bipolar diathermy does not use a patient plate, instead both electrodes are located within the probe held by the surgeon. This type of diathermy is used for neurosurgery and plastic surgery since it uses less power.

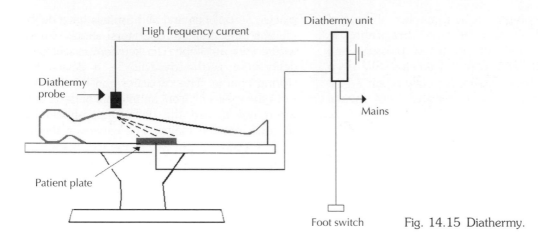

Fig. 14.15 Diathermy.

✂ Activity

There are numerous other ways in which electricity is used diagnostically and therapeutically in hospitals. Find out about the following:
Electromyography (EMG), electroconvulsive therapy (ECT), electrical response audiometry (ERA).

▣▣ Summary

- Electricity is the flow of electrons
- Static electricity is the build-up of electrons
- Dynamic (current) electricity is the flow of electrons
- Ohm's law gives the relationship between potential difference, current and resistance
- Power is the amount of energy used in one second and is measured in watts
- Action potentials occur in nerve cells and the heart and are examples of electricity in the body
- Electricity can kill; safe working procedures should be adopted
- Electricity can be used both diagnostically and therapeutically.

▣▣ Review questions

14.1. If a myelinated neurone had lost or damaged its myelin sheath, how would this affect the rate at which it transmitted nerve impulses?

14.2. Name the major ion responsible for:
   a) the resting membrane potential
   b) the action potential.

14.3. In hospital bathrooms all light switches are 'cord-type' switches, give a reason for this.

14.4. What situations would you advise a patient who has had an artificial pacemaker fitted to avoid?

14.5. Why is the refractory period important to the transmission of nerve impulses?

Further reading

Bray, J.J., Cragg, P.A., MacKnight, A.D.C. & Mills, R.G. (1999). *Lecture Notes on Human Physiology* (4th edn). Blackwell Science Ltd, Oxford.

Parbrook, G.D., Davis, P.D. & Parbrook, E.O. (1995). *Basic Physics and Measurements in Anaesthesia* (4th edn). Butterworth Heinemann, Oxford.

The Franklin Institute Online Home page: http://www.fi.edu/biosci/heart.html

PERIODIC TABLE OF THE ELEMENTS

Key:

Atomic number →	H ← symbol
	Hydrogen ← name
	1.0 ← relative atomic mass

I	II											III	IV	V	VI	VII	O or VIII
																	2 **He** Helium 4.0
3 **Li** Lithium 6.9	4 **Be** Beryllium 9.0											5 **B** Boron 10.8	6 **C** Carbon 12.0	7 **N** Nitrogen 14.0	8 **O** Oxygen 16.0	9 **F** Fluorine 19.0	10 **Ne** Neon 20.2
11 **Na** Sodium 23.0	12 **Mg** Magnesium 24.3											13 **Al** Aluminium 27.0	14 **Si** Silicon 28.1	15 **P** Phosphorus 31.0	16 **S** Sulphur 32.1	17 **Cl** Chlorine 35.5	18 **Ar** Argon 39.9
19 **K** Potassium 39.1	20 **Ca** Calcium 40.0	21 **Sc** Scandium 45.0	22 **Ti** Titanium 47.9	23 **V** Vanadium 50.9	24 **Cr** Chromium 52.0	25 **Mn** Manganese 54.9	26 **Fe** Iron 55.9	27 **Co** Cobalt 58.9	28 **Ni** Nickel 58.7	29 **Cu** Copper 63.5	30 **Zn** Zinc 65.4	31 **Ga** Gallium 69.7	32 **Ge** Germanium 72.6	33 **As** Arsenic 74.9	34 **Se** Selenium 79.0	35 **Br** Bromine 79.9	36 **Kr** Krypton 83.8
37 **Rb** Rubidium 85.5	38 **Sr** Strontium 87.6	39 **Y** Yttrium 88.9	40 **Zr** Zirconium 91.2	41 **Nb** Niobium 92.9	42 **Mo** Molybdenum 95.9	43 **Tc** Technetium 99.0	44 **Ru** Ruthenium 101.1	45 **Rh** Rhodium 102.9	46 **Pd** Palladium 106.4	47 **Ag** Silver 107.9	48 **Cd** Cadmium 112.4	49 **In** Indium 114.8	50 **Sn** Tin 118.7	51 **Sb** Antimony 121.8	52 **Te** Tellurium 127.6	53 **I** Iodine 126.9	54 **Xe** Xenon 131.3
55 **Cs** Caesium 87.0	56 **Ba** Barium 137.3	57 **La** Lanthanium 138.9	72 **Hf** Hafnium 178.5	73 **Ta** Tantalium 181.0	74 **W** Tungsten 183.9	75 **Re** Rhenium 186.2	76 **Os** Osmium 190.2	77 **Ir** Iridium 192.2	78 **Pt** Platinum 195.1	79 **Au** Gold 197.0	80 **Hg** Mercury 200.6	81 **Tl** Thallium 204.4	82 **Pb** Lead 207.2	83 **Bi** Bismuth 209.0	84 **Po** Polonium 210.0	85 **At** Astatine 210.0	86 **Rn** Radon (222.0)
87 **Fr** Francium 223.0	88 **Ra** Radium 226.0	89 **Ac** Actinium 227.0															

58 **Ce** Cerium 140.1	59 **Pr** Praseodymium 140.9	60 **Nd** Neodymium 144.2	61 **Pm** Promethium (147.0)	62 **Sm** Samarium 150.4	63 **Eu** Europium 152.0	64 **Gd** Gadolinium 157.2	65 **Tb** Terbium 158.9	66 **Dy** Dysprosium 162.5	67 **Ho** Holmium 164.9	68 **Er** Erbium 167.3	69 **Tm** Thulium 168.9	70 **Yb** Ytterbium 173.0	71 **Lu** Lutetium 175.0
90 **Th** Thorium 232.0	91 **Pa** Protactinium 231.0	92 **U** Uranium 238.1	93 **Np** Neptunium (237.0)	94 **Pu** Plutonium 239.1	95 **Am** Americium (243.0)	96 **Cm** Curium (247.0)	97 **Bk** Berkelium (247.0)	98 **Cf** Californium (251.0)	99 **Es** Einsteinium (254.0)	100 **Fm** Fermium (253.0)	101 **Md** Mendelevium (256.0)	102 **No** Nobelium (254.0)	103 **Lr** Lawrencium (257.0)

Number in parenthesis ( ) is the mass number of the most stable isotopes.

GLOSSARY

Acceleration The rate at which the velocity of an object changes.

Acid An acid donates hydrogen ions and has a pH below 7.

Acidosis When blood is more acidic than normal, pH less than 7.35.

ADP Adenosine diphosphate.

Aerobic Requires the presence of oxygen.

Aerosol Colloid formed when a solid or liquid is dispersed in a gas.

Alcohol An organic compound containing an OH group. Ethanol is commonly referred to as alcohol.

Alkali A base which dissolves in water giving a solution with a pH above 7.

Alkalosis When blood is more alkaline than normal, pH more than 7.45.

Alleles Different types of the same gene which code for different characteristics.

Alpha particle A particle (helium nucleus) emitted from the nucleus of a radioactive element.

Alveolus (alveoli – pl) Air sac in the lungs where gas exchange occurs.

Amino acid The building block from which proteins are made. Each amino acid molecule has an amino group – NH_2 and also an acid group – COOH.

Anaemia A fall in the concentration of circulating haemoglobin in the blood, reducing the oxygen-carrying capacity of the blood.

Anaerobic Does not require the presence of oxygen.

Analgesic A substance given for pain relief.

Anion A negatively charged ion.

Antibiotic A chemical synthesised by microorganisms which inhibits the growth or kills a different microorganism.

Antibody A protein (immunoglobin) produced in response to foreign bodies entering the body.

Antigen A substance which causes the synthesis of antibodies.

Antigen presenting cell Cells which possess antigens that are expressed on their surface, and together with MHC proteins are recognised by T-cells.

Antioxidant A substance which counteracts the effects of free radicals.

Antipyretic A substance that reduces fever.

Atherosclerosis A condition in which the arteries become narrower from fatty plaque deposits. This results in loss of elasticity and hardening of the arteries.

Atom The smallest part of an element which can take place in a chemical reaction.

ATP Adenosine triphosphate – biological energy carrier.

Atrium (atria – pl) Upper chamber of the heart.

Autosomal dominance A dominant allele, not on a sex chromosome.

Autosome Chromosomes of the same number and type in males and females.

Bacteraemia Bacteria growing in the tissue but detected in blood.

Bacterium (bacteria – pl) Microorganism lacking a true nucleus – DNA is a single molecule free in the cytoplasm.

Base A hydrogen ion acceptor which has a pH above 7.

Beta particle An electron emitted from the nucleus of a radioactive element.

Binary fusion Main method of growth for bacteria. The cell divides into two identical parts.

Blood pressure The pressure exerted by blood on the walls of the blood vessels.

Buffer A chemical solution that resists changes in pH upon the addition of an acid or a base.

Carbohydrates Compounds containing carbon, hydrogen and oxygen only. Sugars, starches, cellulose and glycogen are all carbohydrates.

Carboxylic acid An organic acid which contains the COOH group.

Carrier Person with a single copy of an abnormal gene, which codes for a recessive disorder.

Catalyst A substance which will speed up a chemical reaction, but is not used up during the process.

Cation A positively charged ion.

Cell The smallest unit of life which can survive and reproduce independently.

Cell membrane See plasma membrane.

Centre of gravity The point in a body through which all the forces of gravity acting on that body appear to act.

Chromosome Found in the nucleus of a cell and contains the cell's hereditary information.

Codominance Expression of both alleles in the phenotype.

Codon A group of three bases coding for an amino acid.

Coenzyme Assists enzyme function, typically vitamins.

Colloid Particles which are dispersed in a fluid or solid phase. Particles in a colloid are intermediate in size to those in a solution and a suspension.

Commensal A microorganism which lives in or on the body with no harmful effects.

Compound Formed when two or more elements are chemically joined together.

Concentration The amount of solute dissolved in a given volume of solvent.

Concentration gradient The difference in concentration between two regions.

Condensation The process of a gas changing state into a liquid.

Condensation reaction Loss of water when two small molecules react to form a large molecule.

Conduction (electrical) Flow of electrons.

Conduction (thermal) Transfer of heat energy through a substance from a higher to a lower temperature region.

Conjugation Transfer of genetic material between two bacteria by cell to cell contact.

Constriction Narrowing of an opening, see vasoconstriction.

Convection Transfer of heat energy in a fluid (liquid or gas) by the movement of the fluid itself.

Covalent bond A chemical bond formed by the sharing of electrons.

Cytochromes Electron carriers in cellular respiration.

Cytoskeleton The internal skeleton of the cell, made from microtubules which help to move components around the cell.

Dehydration The loss of water.

Deoxyribonucleic acid (DNA) The genetic material of the cell.

Diastole Relaxation of the heart.

Diathermy Application of heat producing energy source to the body's tissues.

Diffusion The movement of particles from an area of high concentration to an area of low concentration.

Dilation Widening of opening, see vasodilation.

Disinfection A process which destroys or inactivates potentially harmful microorganisms.

DNA See deoxyribonucleic acid.

Doppler effect The change of frequency which appears to occur when a wave source and observer are moving relative to each other.

Earth (earthed, earthing) The conductive connection that forms the route by which electricity flows to earth.

Effort The force that is applied when work is done.

Electrode Conducting rods. Positive electrode is called an anode, negative electrode is called a cathode.

Electrolyte A substance which dissociates in water to produce ions. Due to the ions the solution will conduct electricity.

Electromagnetic radiation Energy in the form of waves which have both electric and magnetic properties.

Electron A particle in the atom. It has a negligible mass and a single negative charge.

Element A collection of the same atoms.

Embryo A stage in development from conception to the 8th week.

Emulsion Colloid formed when one liquid is dispersed as droplets in another liquid.

Endoscopy Examination of the interior of the body by the insertion of a fibre-optic tube.

Endotoxin Toxin which is part of the bacterial cell wall.

Energy The ability to do work.

Enzymes Enzymes are proteins which act as a catalyst. Enzymes are specific in their actions and are most effective at particular temperatures and pH.

Equilibrium The state of balance in a reversible reaction when the rate of the forward and the backward reaction is the same – the reaction appears to have stopped. At equilibrium all the reactants and products are present and their concentrations are all constant. The position of equilibrium can be altered by changing the reaction conditions.

Ergonomics The study of the interactions between humans and machines.

Eukaryotic cell A cell which has a nucleus and membrane-bound organelles – animal, plant, algae and fungi cells.

Evaporation The change of state from a liquid to a gas.

Exotoxin Toxin secreted from bacteria as they grow.

Extracellular fluid All fluid that is located outside the cells.

Facultative anaerobe A bacterium which can grow with or without free oxygen.

Fats See lipids.

Fetus/foetus A stage after the 8th week of development to birth.

Fibrillation Uncoordinated, chaotic beating or quivering of the heart muscle. Ventricular fibrillation may lead to cardiac arrest.

Filtration The use of a membrane to separate particles according to size with the aid of pressure.

Fluid Anything that flows. Can be a gas or a liquid.

Force Something which is capable of influencing the motion of an object.

Free radical A particle having an unpaired electron.

Freezing The change of state from a liquid to a solid.

Frequency The number of oscillations per second in a wave.

Friction A force that resists the movement of one object over another.

Functional group Group of atoms that give organic compounds their chemical properties.

Gamma rays Very high energy ionising radiation emitted by some radioactive elements.

Gas A state of matter in which the particles are able to move independently of each other.

Gene A sequence of DNA that instructs the cell to produce a particular protein.

Genetic code Language that is used by a cell to transfer genetic information.

Genetic screening A process to detect the likelihood of a disease in an individual.

Genetic testing Test used to detect genetic changes.

Genome All the genetic material in the cells of a particular organism.

Genotype The genetic composition of an individual or an individual gene.

Glycoprotein A protein that has a sugar molecule attached.

Glycosuria The presence of glucose in the urine.

Gram stain A differential chemical stain which separates bacteria into groups – Gram positive and Gram negative.

Gravity The force of attraction which exists between any two objects.

Haemoglobin Component of erythrocytes which carries oxygen in the body.

Half-life The time for a radioisotope to decay to half its activity.

Heat A form of energy associated with molecular vibrations.

Heterozygous gene The two alleles which make up a gene are different.

Homeostasis A state of balance (equilibrium) between the internal environment of an organism and the external changing environment.

Homozygous gene The two alleles which make up a gene are the same.

Hormone A chemical messenger which is secreted into the bloodstream by endocrine glands.

Hydrocarbon A compound which only contains carbon and hydrogen.

Hydrogen bond Weak forces of attraction that exist between hydrogen atoms and other atoms such as oxygen and nitrogen.

Hydrolysis The splitting of large molecules into smaller molecules by the reaction with water.

Hydrophilic Water loving.

Hydrophobic Water hating.

Hydrostatic pressure The pressure due to the collision of particles of a liquid with the walls of the container.

Hyperglycaemia High levels of glucose in the blood.

Hyperthermia The condition of abnormally high body temperature.

Hypoglycaemia Low levels of glucose in the blood.

Hypothalamus The area of the brain controlling many functions including hormone and temperature regulation.

Hypothermia The condition of abnormally low body temperature.

Hypoxia Lack of oxygen in tissue.

Immune response The response of the immune system to an antigen.

Immunosuppression General reduction of immune system function which increases the risk of infection.

Indicator A substance which changes colour under different conditions – normally pH.

Inertia The tendency of an object to resist a force which is applied to it.

Inflammation The response of tissues to an infection or injury.

Infrared A region of the electromagnetic spectrum.

Interstitial fluid Fluid that is found between the cells.

Intracellular fluid Fluid found inside cells.

Intravenous Into the vein.

Ion An atom or group of atoms that have an electric charge.

Ionic bond Bonds formed by the loss or gain of electrons. Ions are formed.

Ionising radiation Electromagnetic radiation which has sufficient energy to ionise matter.

Isomers Compounds having the same number of atoms but different structures.

Isotonic A solution that contains the same concentration of solute particles either side of a membrane.

Isotopes Atoms of the same element which have different numbers of neutrons in their nuclei.

Karyotype Arrangement of chromosomes according to size.

Kinetic energy The energy of movement.

Laser Light amplified by stimulated emission of radiation.

Latent heat Additional heat energy required to change the state of a substance.

Lever A machine which enables us to apply a force at one point and see its effect at another.

Lipids Water insoluble organic compounds commonly referred to as fats.

Lipoprotein A protein that has a lipid attached.

Liquid The state of matter in which particles are held together by weak forces.

Liquid crystal A substance that flows like a liquid but maintains some of the ordered structure characteristic of a crystal.

Load The force of resistance that must be overcome when work is done.

Locus Specific site of a gene on a chromosome.

Lubrication A substance that reduces friction between touching surfaces.

Lymph Extracellular fluid located in the lymph vessels.

Lymphatic system System that includes lymph glands where lymphocytes and macrophages are located to filter antigens. Also drains excess fluid from the extracellular space.

Lymphocyte A type of white blood cell.

Macromolecule A very large molecule made up of smaller repeating units.

Magnetic field The region around a magnet or electrical conductor where a magnetic force can be detected.

Major histocompatibility complex (MHC) A group of genes coded for cell surface proteins important in the recognition of antigens by T-cells.

Mass Quantity of matter of an object.

Matter Anything that occupies space and has mass.

Mechanical advantage The ratio of the load divided by effort in a particular machine.

Meiosis Cell division that halves the chromosome number.

Metabolic rate The amount of energy released in the body in a given period of time.

Metabolism The manufacture and breakdown of chemical substances in the body.

Microwave A region of the electromagnetic spectrum.

Mineral Inorganic substance required by the body.

Mitochondrion Cell organelle important in aerobic respiration.

Mitosis Cell division, forming two identical cells.

Molar mass The mass of one mole of substance.

Molar solution A molar solution contains one mole of the dissolved substance in one litre of solution.

Mole A mole is the amount of substance which contains the same number of particles (6×10^{23}) as there are atoms in $12\,g$ of carbon-12.

Molecule Two or more atoms joined together by a covalent bond.

Moment The turning forces about a pivot.

Mucopeptide Unique polysaccharide of bacterial cell walls.

Multifactorial trait Inheritance controlled by many genes plus the effect of the environment.

Mutation A change in the structure of a gene.

Negative feedback Restores homeostasis by acting in a direction opposite to the stimulus or abnormality.

Neutral Solution with pH of 7.

Non-ionising radiation Electromagnetic radiation which does not have sufficient energy to ionise matter.

Nosocomial infection Infections acquired by patients during their stay in hospital.

Nucleic acid Class of organic compounds that include RNA and DNA.

Oedema Accumulation of excess interstitial fluid.

Osmosis The movement of solvent particles across a selectively permeable membrane from an area of high solvent concentration to an area of low concentration.

Osmotic pressure The pressure needed to stop osmosis.

Oxidation The addition of oxygen or loss of electrons.

Partial pressure The pressure exerted by one of the gases present in a mixture of gases.

Particle Any unit of matter – atoms, molecules or ions.

Pathogen A microorganism which harms or damages the body.

Peptide bond The bond formed when two amino acids combine.

pH scale The scale of hydrogen ion concentration with a range from 0 to 14.

Phenotype Physical expression of the genotype.

Phospholipid A lipid that has two fatty acids and a phosphate group and is found in the cell membrane.

Pivot The turning point when a lever is in use.

Plasma The fluid part of the blood.

Plasma membrane A membrane that surrounds the contents of a cell and separates it from its environment.

Plasma proteins The proteins found in the blood, the major one being albumin.

Plasmid Small circular DNA molecule in bacteria, which code for additional genetic information.

Polar A molecule that has slightly charged atoms.

Polygenic trait The combined expression of two or more genes, which have a small additive effect.

Polymer See macromolecule.

Polypeptide A chain of amino acids joined together.

Polysaccharide Many sugar molecules joined together.

Positron A positively charged nuclear particle with the same mass as an electron.

Positive feedback System acts in the direction of change or abnormality.

Potential energy The stored energy.

Pressure The force per unit area acting on a surface.

Products Materials formed during a chemical reaction.

Prokaryotic cell A cell which has no nucleus or membrane-bound organelles.

Proteins Molecules consisting of very long chains of amino acids.

Pulley A grooved wheel with a rope that permits the change of direction of a force.

Punnett square Simple diagrammatic method to predict the outcome of mating.

Pyaemia Bacteria and white cells forming pus in the blood.

Radiation Energy in the form of electro-magnetic waves which is emitted from a source.

Radioactivity The property of some elements to emit ionising radiation from the nuclei of their atoms.

Radiography The recording of photographs of internal body structures by using ionising radiation (X- or gamma rays).

Radioisotope An isotope of an element which emits ionising radiation.

Radiotherapy The treatment of disease by the use of ionising radiation.

Radiowaves A region of the electromagnetic spectrum.

Reactants The substances that take part in a chemical reaction.

Recessive allele The allele which is not expressed unless two copies of it are present in the same gene.

Redox reaction A reaction that involves both reduction and oxidation.

Reduction Addition of hydrogen or the gain of electrons.

Relative atomic mass The relative mass of an atom on a scale where an atom of carbon-12 is 12.000.

Respiration The release of energy from glucose in the cell.

Reversible reaction A reaction that can go both in a forward and a backward direction depending on the conditions.

Ribonucleic acid (RNA) A single stranded nucleic acid important in protein synthesis. Three types: ribosomal RNA (rRNA) found in the ribosomes, messenger RNA (mRNA) which contains the genetic information from DNA as codons, and transfer RNA (tRNA) which binds to mRNA and carries an amino acid during translation.

RNA See ribonucleic acid.

Salt An ionic compound formed when an acid is neutralised by a base.

Septicaemia Bacteria growing in the blood.

Solid The state of matter where the particles have strong forces of attraction between them and the substance has a definite shape.

Solute A substance which dissolves in a solvent, to make a solution.

Solution Uniform distribution of solute particles which are dissolved in solvent.

Solvent A liquid which is used to dissolve substances.

Specific heat capacity The amount of heat needed to raise 1 kg of a substance by 1 °C.

Sphygmomanometer Non-invasive equipment used to measure arterial blood pressure.

States of matter Solid, liquid and gas.

Sterilisation A process which kills all microorganisms.

Stimulus A change in the environment, which the body can detect.

Substrate The substance on which an enzyme acts.

Synovial fluid Lubricating fluid in body joints.

Systole Contraction of the heart.

Temperature A measure of the 'hotness' of a body.

Thermal conductivity A measure of the ability of a substance to conduct heat through itself.

Thermography Detection of disease by the increase in emission of infrared radiation.

Thermometer A device for measuring temperature.

Transcription Formation of RNA from DNA.

Translation Formation of protein from mRNA.

Ultrasound High frequency sound waves.

Ultraviolet A region of the electromagnetic spectrum.

Vacuum A space from which almost all air or gas has been removed.

Vasoconstriction The constriction (narrowing) of blood vessels.

Vasodilation The dilation (widening) of blood vessels.

Vector Any physical quantity that has both magnitude and direction.

Vector (biological) An agent which can carry pathogens from one host to another.

Ventilation Breathing or respiration.

Ventricles Lower chambers of the heart.

Virulence Measure of the ability of a pathogen to produce disease.

Virus Small microorganism composed of an outer protein coat and a single nucleic acid.

Vitamins Organic molecules that are essential to life.

Wavelength The distance between two identical points of adjacent waves.

Weight A measure of the force of attraction of a body to the earth.

Work Transfer of energy from one object to another.

X-rays A region of the electromagnetic spectrum.

ANSWERS

Introduction

Measurements and units

Exercise 0.1:
(a) 34 kg
(b) 100.5 m
(c) 6300 J

Exercise 0.2:
(a) 5×10^{-10}
(b) 3.01×10^8
(c) 7.81×10^7
(d) 1.284×10^5

Exercise 0.3:
(a) 1 mcg
(b) 0.474 kJ
(c) 0.7 or 7×10^{-1}

Exercise 0.4:
(a) 60%, 85%, 36%
(b) 1/25 = 4%; 1/10 = 10%; 1/40 = 2.5%

Exercise 0.5:
Number of measures required = 8 ÷ 10
One measure = 2 mL, so 8 ÷ 10 × 2 = 1.6 mL required

Exercise 0.6:
37.08, expressed to one decimal place this becomes 37.1 °C

Review questions – Measurement and units

Answers to further questions
Maths. 1
Increase in pulse rate = $9 \, \text{min}^{-1}$

$$\% \text{ increase} = \frac{\text{increase in pulse rate}}{\text{resting pulse rate}} \times 100$$
$$= 9 \div 72 = 12.5\%$$

Maths. 2
(a) Polly's body contains 7 ÷ 100 × 50 kg = 3.5 kg blood
Converting to grams, this is equivalent to 3500 g
Percentage of blood given =
$$\frac{\text{Mass of blood given}}{\text{Total body blood mass}} \times 100$$
$$= 600 \div 3500 \times 100\% = 17.1\%$$

(b) Joyce's body mass is 10 stone = 63.5 kg
Joyce's body contains 7 ÷ 100 × 63.5 kg = 4.45 kg blood
Converting to grams, this is equivalent to 4450 g
Percentage of blood given =

$$\frac{\text{Mass of blood given}}{\text{Total body blood mass}} \times 100$$
$$= 600 \div 4450 \times 100\%$$
$$= 13.5\%$$

Maths. 3
Convert the dose required to milligrams (mg)
Dose required = $1.250 \times 10^3 \, \text{mg} = 1250 \, \text{mg}$
Using the formula:

Number of measures to be given
$$= \frac{\text{Dose prescribed}}{\text{Dose per measure}}$$
$$= 1250 \div 250$$
$$= 5 \text{ tablets}$$

Maths. 4
Maximum urine production at 48 min
    After 120 min, 2 mL/min is produced

Chapter 1: Atoms

Exercise 1.1:
Electronic arrangement for lithium:
Li   2, 1

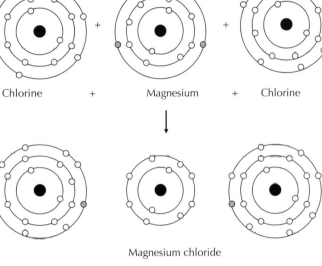

Exercise 1.2:
Electron diagram for the formation of magnesium chloride:

Chlorine   +   Magnesium   +   Chlorine

Magnesium chloride

Exercise 1.3:
Electron diagram for oxygen molecule

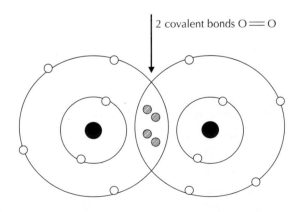

2 covalent bonds O $=$ O

Exercise 1.4:
Calculate the mass of:
a)   0.5 moles of magnesium = 0.5×24.3
        $= 12.15$ g
b)   2 moles of magnesium = 2×24.3
        $= 48.6$ g

Calculate the number of moles of:

a)   64 g of sulphur = $\dfrac{64}{32.1} = 1.99$ mol

b)   0.32 g of sulphur = $\dfrac{0.32}{32.1} = 0.009$ mol

Review questions – Chapter 1: Atoms

1.1.   24 electrons, 24 protons, 27 neutrons

1.2.   a) $C = 12 + (O = 16 \times 2) = 44\,g$
1.2.   b) $C = 12 + (H = 1 \times 4) = 16\,g$
1.2.   c) $(C = 12 \times 12) + (H = 1 \times 22) + (O = 16 \times 11) = 324\,g$

1.3.   a)   Water is covalent
1.3.   b)   Carbon dioxide is covalent
1.3.   c)   Potassium chloride is ionic
1.3.   d)   Haemoglobin is covalent

1.4.   Steam is a gas, water is a liquid. The particles in a gas will have more kinetic energy than particles in water. Therefore when steam comes into contact with skin there is a greater transfer of energy.

1.5.   Iron – ferrum is the Latin name for iron

Chapter 2: Water and electrolytes
Exercise 2.1
Concentration in beaker B

$$\text{number of moles of glucose} = \frac{20}{180} = 0.11$$

$$\text{concentration of glucose} = \frac{0.11}{1} = 0.11\,\text{mol/L}$$

Concentration in beaker C

$$\text{number of moles of glucose} = \frac{200}{180} = 1.11$$

$$\text{concentration of glucose} = \frac{1.11}{1} = 1.11\,\text{mol/L}$$

Exercise 2.2
From Fig. 2.21
1.   The most abundant intracellular cation is potassium
2.   The most abundant extracellular cation is sodium
3.   The most abundant extracellular anion is chloride

Review questions – Chapter 2: Water and electrolytes
2.1.   a) solution b) suspension c) colloid d) suspension.

2.2.   The laxative is not absorbed and is retained within the intestine. This results in a lowering of water concentration in the intestine. Water then flows by osmosis from the surrounding tissue into the intestine. Patients who are taking laxatives should drink fluids to prevent dehydration.

2.3.   Salty snacks increase the concentration of sodium ions in the extracellular fluid. The extracellular fluid becomes hypertonic relative to the intracellular fluid, this triggers the thirst mechanism and the person will then take in fluid – a pint of your best please landlord!

2.4.   a)   Osmosis is the movement of solvent (water) but diffusion is the movement of the solute.

b)   Osmolarity expresses the concentration of a solute in terms of the number of particles it dissociates into in solution. Molarity is the number of moles of solute per litre of solution and it does not take into account whether the solute dissociates.

2.5.   Damage to the capillary walls allows plasma proteins to leak into the interstitial space and into an area where the epidermal layer of the skin has separated due to the rubbing of the shoe. Water moves by osmosis into this area causing a blister.

Chapter 3: Acids and bases
Exercise 3.1:
(a)   The pH of the hydrochloric acid solution is 1.0 pH. Since ethanoic acid is a weak acid it would have a higher pH than hydrochloric acid which is a strong acid.

(b)   The urine sample would have a pH of 0.00001 mol/L.

Exercise 3.2:
pH is low – acidosis
P_{CO_2} is high
$[HCO_3^-]$ is normal
Conclusion – respiratory acidosis

Exercise 3.3:

Review questions – Chapter 3: Acids and bases

3.1.   fruit juice > black coffee > fresh milk > baking soda > soap powder > oven cleaner

3.2.   sodium bicarbonate + stomach acid → sodium chloride + water + carbon dioxide

$NaHCO_3 + HCl \rightarrow NaCl + H_2O + CO_2$

3.3.   pH 7.50 is high – alkalosis
Pco$_2$ is low
[HCO$_3^-$] is normal
Conclusion – respiratory alkalosis

3.4.   When a person is hyperventilating carbon dioxide is being lost from the body due to excessive ventilation. A bag placed over the mouth and nose enables the person to re-inhale the carbon dioxide loss.

3.5.   pH 7.30 is low – acidosis
Pco$_2$ 4.3 is low
[HCO$_3^-$] 18 is low
Metabolic acidosis compensated for by respiratory alkalosis

Chapter 4: Biomolecules
Exercise 4.1
Draw the structures of the amino acids glycine, alanine and phenylalanine

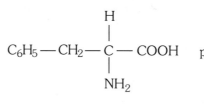

glycine   alanine

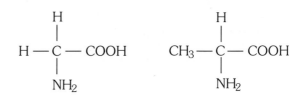

phenylalanine

Exercise 4.2
The other strand of DNA would have the following code   ATTGCTACG

Review questions – Chapter 4: Biomolecules
4.1.

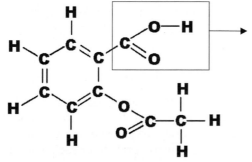

Carboxylic acid functional group

4.2.   The enzymes for protein digestion are secreted in their inactive form to prevent autodigestion. The stomach wall is protected by a mucus lining; however a break in the mucus lining can lead to gastric ulcers due to autodigestion by the enzyme pepsin and hydrochloric acid present in gastric juice.

4.3. Lactose intolerance is due to the lack of the enzyme lactase. Milk contains lactose. However, with yoghurt and cheese the lactose has been fermented to lactic acid, so they can be eaten by people who are lactose intolerant.

4.4. Hormones are proteins and if insulin or growth hormone are given orally, then they would be broken down into their amino acids, before the body could use them.

4.5. a) Storing Clinstix© in the fridge would slow down the rate of reaction of the enzyme, so no colour change should occur within the time limits.

b) Temperatures of above 50°C would denature the enzyme and no colour change would be observed, giving a false reading.

c) The reactant in the Clinstix'© is an enzyme. After its 'shelf life' had expired it would start to decompose and so a false reading would be given.

Chapter 5: Cells
Exercise 5.1
(a) Phenylalanine, glutamine, valine, asparagine.
(b)
(i) No effect in that GUG and GUA both code for valine but threonine would be the next amino acid, not asparagine.
(ii) The first amino acid would be leucine.

Exericse 5.2
1 (ii) chromatid
2 (iv) anaphase
3 (i) cytokinesis
4 (iii) meiosis II

Review questions – Chapter 5: Cells

5.1. Human cells have DNA in a nucleus, membrane-bound organelles, surrounded by a plasma membrane. Bacteria have DNA free in the cytoplasm, no membrane-bound organelles and a cell wall containing mucopeptide.

5.2. Membranes need to be fluid structures to allow molecules to move in and out of the cell.

5.3. Transcription is the copying of DNA into mRNA whereas translation is the synthesis of peptides in the order dictated by the sequence of bases on the mRNA.

5.4. Exocytosis is the movement of intracellular vesicles to the plasma membrane where the membranes fuse and the contents of the vesicle are released to the extracellular space. Endocytosis is the invagination of the plasma membrane around a substance to form an intracellular vesicle. The vesicle can then fuse with a lysosome to destroy the contents of the vesicle.

5.5. Mitosis – to ensure an exact cell replica. Meiosis – to allow the number of chromosomes to remain the same after fertilisation.

5.6. Viruses and prions are not cells because they cannot live independently, i.e. they cannot replicate outside a living cell.

Chapter 6: Genetics
Exercise 6.1
There will be an equal chance of having children with blue or brown eyes.

Review questions – Chapter 6: Genetics

6.1. Phenotype is the expression of genes which are seen in an individual whereas genotype describes the genetic make-up of an individual and can be applied to a pair of single genes or the total number of genes.

6.2. Babies are tested at birth because there is a relatively high incidence in the population and it is possible to treat the disease.

6.3. 1 in 2.

6.4. Epistasis or incomplete penetrance.

6.5. Gene therapy depends on identification and cloning of the defective gene but most importantly requires a vector which will not cause disease and can reach the appropriate cells.

Chapter 7: Microorganisms
Exercise 7.1
32 after 1 hour.

Exercise 7.2

Some products can be used as disinfectants or antiseptics because they are used at different dilutions. Look carefully at the labels and read instructions for use!

Review questions – Chapter 7: Microorganisms

7.1.   Bacteria grow by binary fission, yeast by budding, viruses by using their host cell components to synthesise their own.

7.2.   a) Cross-infection is when an infection results from another person; self-infection is when the infection is caused from a different site on the patient's body.

b)   Sterilisation kills all microorganisms including endospores and viruses; disinfection kills potentially harmful microorganisms.

7.3.   To reduce the risk of contaminating equipment and people.

7.4.   Gram-negative bacteria and *Staphylococcus aureus*.

7.5.   Bacteria can be transmitted through contact – either by contaminated hands or clothing. Chemical disinfection can be used to remove them.

Chapter 8: Immunology
Exercise 8.1

Any condition ending in 'itis', e.g. bronchitis, tonsillitis, appendicitis, colitis.

Exercise 8.2

Immunisation protects the individual and helps to reduce the spread of the disease in the population. Examples such as the incidence of polio today could be given.

Review questions – Chapter 8: Immunology

8.1.   It has antigen binding sites and sites for complement and phagocyte binding which enhance the removal of the antigen from the body.

8.2.   HIV attacks T-helper cells which are needed to mount both cell-mediated and antibody-mediated responses.

8.3.   Adaptive immunity is characterised by its specificity for a particular antigen and memory.

8.4.   Cytokines are chemical soluble molecules produced by cells other than lymphocytes in the immune response.

8.5.   The inflammatory response is characterised by redness, swelling and pain. It is a non-specific response.

8.6.   Immunisation with a vaccine triggers the production of antibodies and memory cells. A second exposure to the vaccine increases the number of antibodies, which are also more specific. If the same pathogen is encountered then the circulating memory cells will be stimulated to produce antibodies within a short time period.

Chapter 9: Fluids
Exercise 9.1

Convert the following to kilopascals
i) $760 \, \text{mmHg} = 760 \div 7.5 = 101.3 \, \text{kPa}$
ii) $120 \, \text{mmHg} = 120 \div 7.5 = 16 \, \text{kPa}$

Convert the following to cmH_2O
i) $0.5 \, \text{kPa} = 0.5 \times 10.5 = 5.3 \, cmH_2O$
ii) $760 \, \text{mmHg} = 760 \times \dfrac{10.2}{7.5} = 1033.6 \, cmH_2O$

Exercise 9.2

Change in intra-alveolar pressure during inspiration $= 100.9 - 101.3 = -0.4 \, \text{kPa}$

Change in intra-alveolar pressure during expiration $= 101.7 - 101.3 = +0.4 \, \text{kPa}$

Change in intrapleural pressure during inspiration $= 100.2 - 101.3 = -1.1 \, \text{kPa}$

Change in intrapleural pressure during expiration $= 101.0 - 101.3 = -0.3 \, \text{kPa}$

Note the intrapleural pressures are always negative, whilst the intra-alveolar pressures can be negative or positive.

Review questions – Chapter 9: Fluids

9.1.   To increase the flow of an enema the nurse can either increase the height of the suspended container or increase the diameter of the tubing.

9.2 $P_{N_2} = \dfrac{79 \times 101.3}{100} = 80.03\,\text{kPa}$

9.3.   At depths nitrogen becomes very soluble in blood – this nitrogen can then form bubbles in the tissue and blood as the diver resurfaces. To avoid this situation helium is used – the solubility of helium in water is much less than that of nitrogen.

9.4.   Each gas will diffuse down its own partial pressure gradient. So oxygen diffuses into the blood and carbon dioxide diffuses into the alveolus.

9.5.   Water is the least viscous, then plasma, blood being the most viscous. Blood contains blood cells whilst plasma contains proteins and water does not contain any particles.

Chapter 10: Nutrition
Exercise 10.1
a)   apples = $150 \div 4.183 = 35.9\,\text{Cal}/100\,\text{g}$
b)   digestive biscuits = $2026 \div 4.183 =$
      $484.3\,\text{Cal}/100\,\text{g}$
c)   chicken = $408 \div 4.183 = 97.5\,\text{Cal}/100\,\text{g}$
Digestive biscuits give the most energy – highest numerical value.

10.5.

Exercise 10.2
$60 \div (1.60 \times 1.60) = 60 \div 2.56 = 23.44$

The woman is the ideal weight.

Review questions – Chapter 10: Nutrition
10.1.   Eating chocolates provides the body with 'quick' energy since they do not need a great deal of digestion. These types of food increase insulin secretion. Potato is a complex carbohydrate and takes longer to digest – this allows the body to store glucose as glycogen.

10.2.   a) muscle contraction;   b) nerve impulses; c) transport of sodium and potassium ions in and out of cell – solute pumping; d) phagocytosis, pinocytosis.

10.3.   Vitamin C is water soluble so is lost to the cooking water. Vitamin D is fat soluble and so is retained within the food.

10.4.   Disease, trauma, etc. can change a person's energy needs. Patients suffering from major burns need more protein and a higher calorific intake since they are forming new tissue. They can be described as being in a hypercatabolic state. Medical patients only need the 'normal' energy requirement since no new tissue is being formed.

gain of hydrogens - reduction

succinic acid

fumaric acid

hydrogens are lost - oxidation

Chapter 11: Electromagnetic radiation
Exercise 11.1
3×10^{15} (300 nm)

Falls within the UVA region

Exercise 11.2
i) Manganese-56

ii) Xenon-131

Review questions – Chapter 11: Electromagnetic radiation
11.1.   i) α.   ii) β.

11.2. $14 \times 3 = 42$ days.

11.3.   PET gives information about the body's function whereas CT provides structural information.

11.4.   CT scan – metal objects will hide parts of required image due to shielding effects of metal. MRI scan – presence of metal will distort magnetic field and hence image produced.

11.5.   Eye protection – sensitivity of the eye to the effects of UV radiation.

Chapter 12: Temperature and heat
Exercise 12.1
Energy required = specific heat capacity $\times$ mass (kg) $\times$ temperature rise
$$= 4.2 \times 70 \times 2 = 588\,\text{kJ}$$

Exercise 12.2
(a)   98.6 °F

(b)   20 °C

(c)   373 K

Exercise 12.3 Precautions required would include:
- Take temperature at the same time of day
- Use the same thermometer each time and exactly the same method.

Review questions – Chapter 12: Temperature and heat
12.1. $0.850 \times 2260\,\text{kJ} = 1921\,\text{kJ}$

12.2.   A clinical thermometer normally has a temperature range between 35 and 42 °C. The temperature of the ward would be approximately 20 °C. In addition, because of its design it is not suitable for continuous reading.

12.3.   Conduction: the vacuum between the glass walls is an excellent insulator. Convection: the movement of any heated air around the inside container will not cause heat loss as it is enclosed. No convection currents will occur in the vacuum between the glass walls. Radiation losses are minimised by the use of shiny surfaces, inside and out. These reflect the heat rays rather than absorbing them.

12.4.   Avoid where possible medications that may cause problems with thermoregulation or accelerate the possibility of dehydration. Inform the patient or family members of the heat-related risks faced by older patients in hot conditions due to over-exertion or prolonged periods in hot conditions. Make the patient aware of suitable clothing and hydration methods during heat waves. For example, loose-fitting, light-coloured, cotton clothing and drinking extra water.

Chapter 13: Forces and mechanics
Exercise 13.1
A weight of 70 kg exerts a downward force of $70 \times 10\,\text{N} = 700\,\text{N}$

Pressure on area of $0.01\,\text{m}^2$ = force/area = $700 \div 0.01 = 70\,000\,\text{Nm}^{-2}$

A weight of 700 kg exerts a downward force of $700 \times 10\,\text{N} = 7000\,\text{N}$

Pressure on area of $0.1\,\text{m}^2$ = force/area = $7000 \div 0.1 = 70\,000\,\text{Nm}^{-2}$

The pressure is equal in both cases!

Exercise 13.2
The turning force is given by the force multiplied by its distance from the pivot. The weight of father and child can be converted into the downward force in Newtons by multiplying by 10. Hence:

Turning force produced by father = $60 \times 10 \times 1 = 60\,\text{Nm}$ (Newton metres)

Turning force produced by child = $30 \times 10 \times 2 = 60\,\text{Nm}$

The turning forces are equal (and opposite) so the see-saw will balance.

Exercise 13.3

The scissors are an example of a first order lever.
The forceps are an example of a third order lever.

Review questions – Chapter 13: Forces and mechanics

13.1.   Only a small force is needed to keep the trolley moving. It is already moving so the only significant force to be overcome is friction. You come to a corner and you find that more force is needed to get it round the corner. To move the trolley in a new direction an additional force in that direction must be applied.

13.2.   Your feet should provide a wide base whilst lifting so as to ensure that the body's centre of gravity falls within that base throughout the lifting manoeuvre. If not, you are likely to topple over!

13.3.   The introduction of a liquid between the surfaces will reduce the friction. The intermolecular forces between molecules in a liquid are sufficiently weak such that the molecules of a liquid are able to roll over each other whereas those of a solid are not.

13.4.   Holding a box at arm's length is more tiring than holding it close to your body. Consider the arm and the load to be a 3rd order lever. Increasing the distance of the load from the pivot (elbow or shoulder) will increase the turning force so the load will appear heavier since the downward force will be increased.

Chapter 14: Electricity
Exercise 14.1
How much current does a 60 watt electric light bulb use on a 240 V mains supply?

Power (W) = voltage (V) × current (A)
$$\frac{0.8 \times 1000}{5} = 160$$

Exercise 14.2
a)   0.8 seconds
b)   60 ÷ 0.8 = 75 beats per minute
c)   nerve impulse is 5 ms – therefore a nerve impulse is transmitted 160 times faster than a heart beat. $\frac{0.8 \times 1000}{5} = 160$

Review questions – Chapter 14: Electricity
14.1.   Myelin sheath damage will result in short-circuiting of the impulse so that the impulse travels slower and slower; conduction may stop.

14.2.   a)   potassium ion
        b)   sodium ion

14.3   If a normal light switch was used then there is a risk of shock or electrocution since wet skin provides little resistance to the passage of current. The dry cord is an insulator and prevents the passage of any current.

14.4   Patients with pacemakers can experience interference from external electromagnetic fields. There are numerous sources, e.g. anti-theft devices in shops and libraries and microwave ovens. Patients may experience dizziness and syncope.

14.5   The refractory period is a time when the nerve cell will not respond to a stimulus. This means that the action potential has to move in one direction.

INDEX